AF884601

CDN Study Guide 2025-2026

Complete Review + 450 Test Questions and Detailed Answer Explanations for the Certified Dialysis Nurse Exam (3 Full-Length Exams)

Copyright 2025 by Newstone Test Prep - All rights reserved.

Printed in the United States of America

Newstone Test Prep is not affiliated with any official testing organization. All test names and registered trademarks belong to the owners or related official testing organizations. Newstone Test Prep does not endorse any political or religious statement via this publication.

This book is geared towards providing precise and reliable information about the topic. This publication is sold with the idea that the publisher is not required to render any accounting, officially or otherwise, or any other qualified services. If further advice is necessary, contacting a legal and/or financial professional is recommended.

From a Declaration of Principles that was accepted and approved equally by a Committee of the American Bar Association and a Committee of Publishers' Associations.

In no way is it legal to reproduce, duplicate, or transmit any part of this document, either by electronic means, or in printed format. Recording this publication is strictly prohibited, and any storage of this document is not allowed unless with written permission from the publisher. All rights reserved.

The information provided herein is stated to be truthful and consistent, in that any liability, in terms of inattention or otherwise, by any usage or abuse of any policies, processes, or directions contained within, is the solitary and utter responsibility of the recipient reader. Under no circumstances will any legal responsibility or blame be held against the publisher for any reparation, damages, or monetary loss due to the information herein, either directly or indirectly.

Respective authors own all copyrights not held by the publisher.

The information herein is offered for informational purposes solely, and is universally presented as such. The information herein is also presented without contract or any type of guarantee or assurance.

The trademarks presented are done so without any consent, and this publication of the trademarks is without permission or backing by the trademark owners. All trademarks and brands within this book are thus for clarifying purposes only and are owned by the owners themselves, and are not affiliated otherwise with this document.

Table of Contents

Abbreviations

DNA - Deoxyribonucleic acid

PCR - Polymerase chain reaction

HSV - Herpes simplex virus

VZV - Varicella zoster virus

CMV - Cytomegalo virus

MRSA - Methicillin resistant staph aureus

TMP-SMX - Trimethoprim-sulfamethoxazole

UTI - Urinary tract infection

PCP - Pneumocystis jirovecii pneumonia

HCV - Hepatitis C virus

HBV - Hepatitis B virus

HBsAg - Hepatitis B surface antigen

ALT - Alanine transaminase

CNI - Calcineurin inhibitor

ECG - Electrocardiography

CVP - Central venous pressure

PRN - Per need

SGOT - Serum glutamic-oxaloacetic transaminase

SGPT - Serum glutamic pyruvic transaminase

LDH - Lactate dehydrogenase

ALP - Alkaline phosphatase

KDIGO - kidney disease: improving global outcomes

Chapter 1: Physiology of the Kidney

The kidneys' primary function is urine formation. The kidneys also excrete wastes, maintain fluid and electrolyte balance, maintain acid-base balance, produce hormones, and regulate blood pressure.

Excretion of Waste Products

Kidneys excrete unwanted waste products, which are formed during metabolic activities in the body. These include urea, which is generated from amino acid metabolism; uric acid, which is generated from nucleic acid metabolism; creatinine, which is generated from muscle tissue metabolism; bilirubin, which is generated from the degradation of hemoglobin; and other substances such as drugs and toxins.

Maintenance of Water Balance

Through the anti-diuretic hormone, also known as vasopressin, the kidneys retain water when it is depleted and excrete it when it is excessive.

Maintenance of Electrolyte Balance

The maintenance of sodium-specific electrolyte balance is related to water balance. When the body water osmolarity drops, the kidneys store sodium; when it rises, they remove it.

Maintenance of Acid–Base Balance

The pH of the blood and other bodily fluids should be kept within a certain range. It is accomplished by renal function, and because so many acids are produced during metabolic processes, the body is always in danger of developing acidosis. Thus, the kidneys, lungs, and blood buffers remove these acids. The kidneys are one of the main organs that help avoid acidosis. The kidneys also excrete some metabolic acids, such as sulfuric and phosphoric acids.

Hemopoietic/ Thrombopoietic Function

Erythropoietin, a stimulating factor produced by the kidneys, stimulates erythropoiesis in the bone marrow. Thrombopoietin stimulates the production of thrombocytes (platelets) and is produced by the liver.

Endocrine Function

Other hormones secreted by the kidneys, apart from erythropoietin and thrombopoietin, are renin and prostaglandins.

Blood Pressure Regulation

This is achieved through two mechanisms: the renin-angiotensin-aldosterone system and the extracellular fluid volume regulation.

Regulation of Blood Calcium Level

The kidneys convert vitamin D into its active form. When activated, vitamin D helps absorb calcium from the intestines. Vitamin D3 is an active and important form of vitamin D that is synthesized in the skin from 7-dehydrocholesterol by ultraviolet rays from the sunlight. It is then converted into 25-hydroxycholecalciferol in the liver, and finally into 1, 25-dihydroxycholecalciferol in the kidney.

External Structure of the Kidney

Healthy adult kidneys are paired, reddish-brown organs that typically measure about 10–12 cm long, 5–6 cm wide, and 2–3 cm deep. Each kidney has about 1–1.3 million nephrons. The kidneys lie retroperitoneally at the level of the T12–L3 vertebrae on each side of the vertebral column and in the posterior abdominal wall. The kidneys lie deep to the 11th and 12th ribs. They move 2–3 cm vertically with the movement of the diaphragm, which occurs when we breathe.

The kidney has anterior and posterior surfaces, medial and lateral margins, and superior and inferior poles. A vertical cleft on the medial margin of each kidney is called the hilum. The hilum serves as an entry and exit point to a space within the kidney called the renal sinus.

Each kidney is surrounded by three main layers: renal fascia, adipose capsule, and the renal capsule from the outer to inner layers. The renal fascia is a layer of connective tissue that provides structural support. It also attaches the kidney to the abdominal wall. The adipose capsule is a pad of fat surrounding the kidney. It protects the kidneys from trauma and helps maintain the position of the kidneys within the abdominal cavity. The renal capsule is a connective tissue that maintains the kidney’s structural integrity and shape and protects its tissue.

Due to the position of the liver on the right part of the abdominal cavity, the right kidney is typically shorter, lighter, and slightly lower than the left.

Blood Supply of the Kidney

The kidneys receive their blood supply from the renal arteries, which are branches of the abdominal aorta. The blood vessels in the kidneys are extremely specialized to support the kidneys in urine formation. Both kidneys receive about 25% of the cardiac output.

The renal artery divides into many segmental arteries after entering the kidney through the hilum, which gives rise to segmental arteries. The segmental artery further subdivides into interlobar arteries that pass into the medulla between the medullary pyramids to form the arcuate arteries. The arcuate artery gives rise to interlobular arteries, from which afferent arterioles arise.

Lymphatic Drainage

The kidney's lymphatic vessels drain into the aorto-caval lymph nodes to the thoracic and then into the venous circulation.

Nerve Supply

The nerve supply to the kidneys comes from the plexus of the renal nerve. It is composed of the parasympathetic and sympathetic fibers of the autonomic nervous system.

Internal Structure of the Kidney

The kidney is composed of three layers, namely, the cortex, medulla, and the renal sinus. The cortex is the outer portion of the kidney. It is dark and granular in appearance and contains the renal corpuscles and convoluted tubules, which may extend into the inner medulla. The medulla is the inner part of the kidney that contains tubular structures and blood vessels arranged in parallel. The renal sinus is occupied by the renal pelvis, calices, blood vessels, nerves, and fat. These structures enter and exit the renal sinus through the hilum.

Microstructure Of the Kidney

The Nephron

The nephron is the functional unit of the kidneys. Each healthy human kidney has about 1–1.3 million nephrons. Each nephron consists of the renal corpuscle, the proximal convoluted tubule, the loop of Henle, the distal convoluted tubule, and the collecting ducts.

Renal Corpuscle

The renal corpuscle is formed by the glomerulus and the Bowman capsule. the glomerulus is a tuft of capillaries with a total area of 0.8 m^2. Enclosed by the Bowman capsule is a cup-like tubule that encloses the glomerulus.

The renal corpuscle is responsible for the filtration of blood through the filtration membrane, which is made up of three layers: the glomerular capillary endothelium, the basement membrane, and the podocyte layer. The basement membrane allows the passage of free and neutral substances that are up to 4 nm in diameter.

Blood comes into the glomerulus through the afferent arteriole, which is a branch of the renal artery, and leaves through the efferent arteriole. The differences in the diameter of the afferent and efferent arterioles causes increased pressure within the glomerular capillary. It also restricts the outward flow of blood from the glomerulus, together with the permeability of the capillaries within the glomerulus to water, electrolytes, and other solutes. This results in a fast and efficient filtration process.

Proximal Convoluted Tubule

The proximal convoluted tubule is the coiled initial portion of the nephron that arises from the Bowman capsule and continues as a descending limb of the loop of Henle. It is about 14 mm long and 55 μm in diameter, and is formed by a layer of cuboidal epithelium that interdigitates and possesses hairlike projections called microvilli.

The primary role of the proximal convoluted tubule is to reabsorb water and electrolytes such as sodium, chlorine, calcium, potassium, and bicarbonates from the renal corpuscular filtrate. Only the proximal convoluted tubule of the nephron can allow the reabsorption of glucose. Any excess glucose beyond the proximal convoluted tubule is removed in the urine.

From the renal corpuscle, the filtrate passes into the proximal convoluted tubule, where about 70% and 80% of water and bicarbonates, respectively, are absorbed at this region from the filtrate. Balance in the reabsorption of bicarbonate ions and the release of hydrogen ions greatly influences the management of the body's acid-base balance.

Loop of Henle

The Loop of Henle consists of the descending limb, hairpin bend, and the ascending limb. The descending limb has one segment: the thin descending segment, which is a continuation of the proximal convoluted tubule. The loop then continues as the ascending limb, which has a thin ascending segment and a thick ascending segment. The thick descending segment has a length of 6 mm and a diameter of 55 μ. It is formed by brush-border cuboidal epithelial cells with multiple mitochondria and descends into the renal medulla. The thin descending segment is formed by flattened epithelial cells without a brush border and continues as the hairpin bend of the loop of Henle. It continues as the ascending limb of the loop of Henle, which also has a thin ascending segment and a thick ascending segment.

Distal Convoluted Tubule

The thick ascending segment of the loop of Henle continues as the distal convoluted tubule. The distal convoluted tubule is about 14–15 mm in length with a diameter of 22–50 μ and is lined by a layer of cuboidal epithelium called intercalated cells.

Collecting Duct

The distal convoluted tubule continues as the collecting duct with a length of 20–22 mm and a diameter of about 40 and 200 μ. It is lined by two types of cuboidal epithelia: the principal or *P* cells and the intercalated cells.

Juxtaglomerular Apparatus

The juxtaglomerular apparatus is a combination of structures situated near the glomerulus of each nephron. It is formed by the macula densa, the mesangial cells, and the juxtaglomerular cells.

The macula densa are cuboidal cells aggregated at the terminal portion of the thick ascending segment of the loop of Henle, just before opening into the distal convoluted tubule and between the afferent and efferent arterioles. The mesangial cells are located in the same region as the macula densa cells. It is also found between glomerular capillaries, where they exert a contractile activity, and which regulates glomerular filtration. Glomerular mesangial cells secretes prostaglandins and cytokines. The juxtaglomerular cells are smooth muscle cells that contain secretory granules within their cytoplasm. It is present in the tunica media and tunica adventitia of the afferent arteriole, shortly before entering the Bowman capsule.

Functions of Juxtaglomerular Apparatus

The juxtaglomerular apparatus secretes hormones, which include renin and prostaglandins. It also regulates the glomerular blood flow and filtration rate. Renin is a hormone released by the juxtaglomerular cells of the juxtaglomerular apparatus. It forms a hormone cascade with angiotensin, which maintains blood pressure. Its release is stimulated by a fall in arterial blood pressure, reduced extracellular fluid volume, reduced sodium chloride concentration, and accelerated sympathetic activity.

Renin catalyzes the conversion of angiotensinogen to angiotensin I, which is physiologically inactive. Angiotensin I is then converted to angiotensin II by an angiotensin-converting enzyme produced in the lungs. Angiotensin II is the most active form of angiotensin. It is a potent arteriolar vasoconstrictor that increases blood pressure by vasoconstriction. It stimulates the release of noradrenaline, also from postganglionic sympathetic fibers with resultant increased blood pressure.

The release of aldosterone from the adrenal cortex is also stimulated by angiotensin II, which causes increased sodium retention that results in increased blood pressure. Angiotensin II constricts the efferent arteriole, which results in increased glomerular filtration rate. The baroreceptor reflex, which is responsible for decreasing the blood pressure, is inhibited by angiotensin II. This increases the blood pressure.

Urine Formation

Urine formation is a complex process involving a series of interrelated events and processes, which are glomerular filtration, tubular reabsorption, and tubular secretion. The adult kidneys make about 1–2 L of urine per day after undergoing these processes, although individual variations may occur.

Processes of Urine Formation

The process of urine formation starts with glomerular filtration, where blood from the afferent arteriole passes through glomerular capillaries, where it is then filtered into the Bowman capsule. The filtrate flows from the Bowman capsule to the tubular portion of the nephron, where the filtrate undergoes changes in both quantity and quality through reabsorption and secretion processes.

Most substances desired by the body, such as water, electrolytes, glucose, and amino acids, are reabsorbed from the filtrate in the tubules. Substances not desired by the body are secreted into the tubule from peritubular blood vessels.

Glomerular Filtration

Glomerular filtration is the first step in the formation of urine. It involves the filtration of blood across the filtration membrane, which is made up of glomerular capillary membrane, basement membrane, and the visceral layer of the Bowman capsule.

The glomerular capillary membrane is made up of a layer of endothelial cells attached to the basement membrane and has fenestrations with a diameter of about 0.1 μ. The basement membrane is formed by the fusion of the endothelium of glomerular capillaries and the epithelium of the Bowman's capsule. The visceral layer of the Bowman capsule is a layer of flattened epithelium that rests on the basement membrane by the extension of their cytoplasm, which gives rise to the pedicle or foot process, with slitlike spaces in between.

The plasma is filtered into the Bowman capsule as blood flows through the glomerular capillaries. All of the plasma's components are filtered, including most plasma proteins, but larger proteins like albumin are normally not filtered. The glomerular filtrate includes all of the plasma components except for plasma proteins.

The glomerular filtration rate (GFR) is defined as the total quantity of filtration formed in all the nephrons of both the kidneys in the given unit of time. Normal glomerular filtration rate is 125 mL per minute.

Tubular Reabsorption

This is the process by which water and other substances are taken up by renal tubular cells from the glomerular filtrate in the renal tubules into the renal medulla interstitial fluid, to the peritubular capillaries, and subsequently back to the blood. This brings about changes in both quality and quantity of the glomerular filtrate as it flows through the tubular portion of the nephron, where a large volume of water, electrolytes, and other substances are reabsorbed.

Reabsorption across the tubular cells occurs by two transport mechanisms: active reabsorption and passive reabsorption. In active reabsorption, molecules move against the electrochemical or concentration gradient, which requires energy. This is commonly seen with reabsorption of molecules such as glucose, sodium, amino acids, potassium, phosphates, sulphates, uric acid, ketones, bicarbonate, and calcium. Passive reabsorption is the transport of molecules along the concentration and electrochemical gradient. This process does not need energy. Examples of such molecules are chloride and urea.

Reabsorption of molecules from the renal tubular lumen to the peritubular capillary occurs through the transcellular route, where the molecules move through the cells lining the tubules. About 88% of the filtrate is reabsorbed in the proximal convoluted tubule. Molecules absorbed from this region include amino acids, glucose, sodium, potassium, bicarbonates, chlorides, phosphates, urea, uric acid, water, and calcium.

The loop of Henle is a major site for reabsorption of sodium and chloride. Sodium, calcium, bicarbonate, and water are reabsorbed at the distal convoluted tubule.

Important Substance Reabsorption

Reabsorption of Sodium

About 70% of sodium in the glomerular filtrate is absorbed from the proximal convoluted tubule, whereas the remaining 30% is absorbed at the collecting duct. Sodium is transported from the glomerular filtrate into the tubular cells, then to the interstitial fluid, and finally into the blood. Sodium is transported at different levels through varying mechanisms. In the proximal convoluted tubule, sodium is exchanged for hydrogen ions in a process called the antiport transport by a sodium counterport protein. Sodium is also transported along with other molecules such as glucose and amino acids by a process known as symport transport by a sodium co-transport protein.

Reabsorption of Water

The reabsorption of water occurs at different points, such as the proximal convoluted tubule, distal convoluted tubule, and the collecting duct, with varying degrees of permeability depending on the segment. Water reabsorption in the proximal convoluted tubule follows the reabsorption of sodium as sodium creates an osmotic gradient, which results in osmosis of water.

The distal convoluted tubule and the collecting duct are normally not permeable to water; however, they become permeable to water in the presence of an antidiuretic hormone. The reabsorption of water from these regions occurs through facultative reabsorption. It depends on the activity of the antidiuretic hormone, which stimulates the water channels known as aquaporins to increase water reabsorption.

Reabsorption of Glucose

Glucose is reabsorbed completely from the proximal convoluted tubule and is transported through a sodium co-transport mechanism, where sodium and glucose are transported by a sodium-dependent glucose co-transporter 2 into the tubular cells. The renal threshold for glucose is 180 mg/dL in venous blood, so higher glucose concentrations are not reabsorbed but excreted in the urine.

Reabsorption of Bicarbonates

Bicarbonate usually exists as sodium bicarbonate in the renal filtrate. It is reabsorbed actively in the form of bicarbonate ions (HCO_3^-) from the proximal convoluted tubule. After the dissociation of sodium bicarbonate into sodium and bicarbonate, the bicarbonate ions are reabsorbed into the bloodstream.

Reabsorption of Amino Acids

Just like glucose, amino acids are also completely reabsorbed from the proximal convoluted tubule along with sodium through a secondary active transport mechanism.

Tubular Secretion

Tubular secretion involves the transport of molecules from the blood into renal tubules. Examples include drugs such as penicillin, derivatives of amino acids, and acids such as 5-hydroxy indole acetic acid and para-aminohippuric acid. Different parts of the renal tubule secrete different molecules and substances. Molecules and substances secreted at the proximal convoluted tubules include potassium, ammonia, and hydrogen ions, whereas those at distal convoluted tubules are potassium, minimal hydrogen ions, and also urea at the loop of Henle.

Chapter 2: Etiologies of Kidney Disease

Diabetes mellitus

Diabetes is one of the most common causes of kidney disease. The high prevalence of diabetes has significantly contributed to the increased prevalence of renal disease.

Chronic hyperglycemia contributes to renal disease in a variety of ways, which include the excess release of free radicals, profibrotic mediators, and proinflammatory cytokines. However, the single most important factor that gives rise to diabetic renal disease is the renin-angiotensin system (RAS). Elevated levels of renin and aldosterone precipitate numerous physiological effects, which include increased sodium reabsorption, vasoconstriction of efferent arterioles, and amplified glomerular capillary permeability. Research has also identified a protein called endothelin-1, which is upregulated in diabetic patients. This protein promotes renal cellular proliferation, podocyte damage, and tissue fibrosis. Excess glucose levels also bind to free amino acids, which create advanced glycation end products (AGEs). When AGEs accumulate and crosslink with collagen, they cause microvascular complications within the kidneys.

All of these factors can lead to significant changes in the physiology of the kidneys, including alterations in glomerular permeability, thickening of the glomerular basement membrane, and an increase in glomerular filtration rate (glomerular hyperfiltration). Over time, this may progress to chronic kidney disease (CKD) and end-stage renal disease (ESRD).

The main goal in the management of diabetic kidney disease is to prevent progression to ESRD. Therefore, the goals of treatment revolve around the control of glycemia and other factors that contribute to kidney disease. Note that a significant proportion of patients with type 1 diabetes and notable microalbuminuria will progress to clinical nephropathy within ten to fifteen years.

Healthcare professionals should aim to control high blood glucose, but this should be done carefully to avoid hypoglycemia. As a general guideline, clinicians often aim for an HbA1c of around 7.0%, although individualized treatment goals may be appropriate based on the clinical manifestations and laboratory results of patients. This goal can be adjusted based on the clinical manifestations and biological results of patients.

If a diabetic patient has concurrent blood hypertension, the anti-hypertensive drug of choice is angiotensin-converting enzyme (ACE) inhibitor. There is concrete evidence that ACE inhibitors slow down the progression of kidney disease in diabetics with high blood pressure. Statins may also be helpful in the prevention of chronic kidney disease since they reduce serum levels of AGEs in diabetic patients.

Diabetics with eGFR below 60 ml/min/1.73m2 can usually continue to take metformin, but if eGFR drops below 30 ml/min/1.73m2, metformin should generally be avoided. Healthcare professionals should closely monitor and adjust the doses of other anti-diabetes drugs according to eGFR levels. Healthcare professionals should pay close attention to the doses of other anti-diabetes drugs according to eGFR levels.

In some cases, patients with diabetes may present with atypical signs and symptoms of renal impairment, such as rapid GFR decline, heavy proteinuria, and active urine sediment. It is vital to seek nephrology referral to optimize patient care, especially for stage 4 CKD.

Blood hypertension

The incidence and prevalence of hypertension (high blood pressure) are extremely high, which predisposes patients to an array of complications such as chronic kidney disease. Some well-documented factors that contribute to the progression of chronic kidney disease (CKD) include fluid overload, fluid retention, upregulated sympathetic nervous system activity, dysfunctional endothelial autoregulation, and the renin-angiotensin-aldosterone system (RAAS).

Hypernatremia and fluid retention

Renal function maintains sodium and fluid balance through regulation of the reabsorption and excretion rates based on hemodynamic changes in the efferent arterioles of the glomeruli. Impaired kidney function may upregulate the reabsorption of sodium and fluids, which can lead to progressive hypernatremia (elevated sodium levels) and edema. Furthermore, elevated sodium intake can significantly contribute to high blood pressure in patients with CKD. The regulation of dietary sodium intake becomes impaired as renal function declines. Some sources refer to this phenomenon as salt sensitivity. Chronically elevated sodium intake promotes arterial stiffness, upregulates the release of proinflammatory cytokines, and reduces the release of nitric oxide (NO).

RAAS activation

The RAAS is a critical regulator of blood pressure that responds to changes in dietary sodium intake. There is concrete evidence that inappropriate RAAS activation may be a contributing factor to kidney disease associated with blood hypertension. Individuals with chronic kidney disease have high plasma renin and angiotensin II levels, which further worsens sodium retention and blood pressure. Research has also found that high angiotensin II production plays a role in the loss of kidney function.

Upregulated sympathetic nervous system activity

The sympathetic nervous system plays a major role in the control of renal function and BP. CKD is associated with overactivity of the sympathetic nervous system. Increased renal sympathetic activity increases renin secretion, tubular sodium reabsorption, and vascular constriction. These effects contribute to hypertension.

Endothelial dysfunction

The endothelium typically produces nitric oxide (NO) to dilate blood vessels. Blood hypertension may cause endothelial dysfunction and further increase the risk of chronic kidney disease. Some factors that give rise to endothelial dysfunction are oxidative stress, high levels of asymmetric and symmetric dimethylarginine, and L-arginine deficiency. Endothelial dysfunction augments the risk of blood hypertension, which causes kidney disease. The latter may also contribute to blood hypertension exacerbation. This creates a vicious cycle that is challenging to manage.

Glomerulonephritis

Glomerulonephritis (GN) is a prevalent etiology of renal failure. It accounts for up to 15% of end-stage renal disease in the United States. Without proper intervention, GN rapidly leads to a high rate of morbidity and mortality. After diabetes and blood hypertension, glomerulonephritis is the third most common cause of ESRD in the U.S.

A subset of patients with glomerulonephritis present with nephritis syndrome, which is associated with a more rapid progression to ESRD. In fact, patients may develop ESRD within weeks of the beginning of nephritic syndrome. Other clinical signs and symptoms of GN include blood hypertension, hematuria, and proteinuria. When GN causes severe damage to podocytes, massive proteinuria and lower extremity edema may follow due to nephrotic syndrome. Despite the value of these clinical signs in the diagnosis of GN, they are rarely helpful in the identification of the specific GN subtype. Therefore, specialists may opt for kidney biopsy to study the pathological lesions and determine the GN subtype.

The management of GN focuses on addressment of the underlying cause. In some cases, GN may be primary, which requires supportive care and a few specific therapies. The prognosis of patients with GN essentially depends on the timing of medical intervention. In general, there are two modalities of therapy in GN. Initially, specific management uses immunosuppressive drugs, such as corticosteroids, rituximab, cyclophosphamide, and plasma exchange. The choice of these drugs depends on disease severity and progression, histological diagnosis, and comorbidities. As GN progresses to chronic kidney disease, other therapeutic modalities are justified, which include regular renal function tests, urine protein excretion rate, and serum albumin. Diet counseling has also proved effective in prevention of fluid overload and electrolyte imbalances.

Maintenance of controlled blood pressure is also important to slow down the progression to ESRD. Loop diuretics, such as furosemide, aid in the removal of fluids and the management of blood pressure. ACE inhibitors and angiotensin receptor blockers (ARBs) are useful in patients with GN who also have diabetes. Severe hypertension or refractory cases may benefit from nitroprusside or other vasodilators.

Finally, healthcare providers should manage the complications that arise due to GN, such as anemia, metabolic acidosis, cardiovascular disease, osteoporosis, and restless leg syndrome.

Polycystic kidney disease

Polycystic kidney disease is an autosomal dominant disease that presents with renal enlargement and cyst formation. Other organ systems may also be affected, which include the liver, spleen, and pancreas. Autosomal dominant polycystic kidney disease (ADPKD) is responsible for 8% of renal failure cases, which makes it the leading genetic cause of ESRD. Although cysts are visible on ultrasound imaging in utero, the symptoms of polycystic kidney disease do not manifest until the third decade of life. About half the patients with ADPKD require a kidney transplant by the age of sixty years.

The clinical presentation of polycystic kidney disease includes pain, blood hypertension, blood in the urine, and damage to the parenchyma of the kidneys. When the cysts get infected or bleed, patients will present with acute renal pain. In addition, recurrent urinary tract infections (UTIs) may be the first presenting sign of ADPKD. This can manifest as bladder infections, acute pyelonephritis, and perinephric abscesses. Additionally, up to a fifth of patients will be affected by renal lithiasis.

Autoimmune diseases

Autoimmune diseases comprise another prominent etiology of kidney disease. These diseases cause renal damage due to the tissue-degrading process mediated by autoantibodies. These molecules generally target the glomeruli, which activates a state of inflammation that gradually causes fibrosis and reduces the number of functional renal units.

Some clinicians may not attempt to differentiate between autoimmune and inflammatory diseases in the context of kidney disease. The most common autoimmune processes that cause renal disease are systemic lupus erythematosus, membranous nephropathy, and renal vasculitis (ANCA-positive). On the other hand, inflammatory diseases include IgG4-related ailments and hemophagocytic processes. In these conditions, there is a generalized inflammation that affects multiple organs, with a special tropism to the kidneys. One condition that causes kidney disease with poorly understood pathophysiology is Henoch Schönlein purpura. This condition is a vasculitis that is mediated by IgA. To remember Henoch Schönlein purpura, think of the mnemonic PAAN (non-blanching purpura, abdominal pain, arthralgia, and nephropathy).

Heavy metal poisoning

Heavy metals poisoning can be acute or chronic dependent on the rate of ingestion. If the metals are ingested chronically through food, water, and skin contact, it usually takes years to cause any damage. Conversely, the inhalation of heavy metals through fumes or dust may cause acute poisoning. Pediatric patients are more prone to accidental ingestion of heavy metals. Surprisingly, barium use and direct injection of gallium during imagery procedures may expose patients to heavy metal poisoning.

Target organs of heavy metals include the central nervous system, liver, lungs, and kidneys. The capacity of the kidneys to reabsorb ions and metals makes them particularly susceptible to parenchymal damage. The type of metal and its duration of exposure play vital roles in the determination of the significance of renal impairment. Initially, heavy metal toxicity can cause acute kidney injury. Without appropriate intervention, it may eventually progress to chronic kidney disease.

Toxicity tests may reveal two patterns of heavy metals in plasma. The first is protein-bound and the second exists in the ionized form. Subsequently, the metals are either excreted from the body or sequestered by the renal tissue. The proximal tubule generally contains both forms of the heavy metals (e.g., bound and free forms). During chronic exposure to heavy metals, the protein-bound form is conjugated by glutathione and metallothionein and is released into the blood. After being reabsorbed by the kidneys, they can cause low-grade inflammation, fibrosis, and kidney failure.

The glomeruli have a different site of reabsorption during acute heavy metal toxicity. This includes the apical membrane of the proximal tubule and the loop of Henle. Acute kidney injury caused by ionized metals triggers cellular death via apoptotic signals (e.g., reactive oxygen species, cytokines).

Drug-induced nephrotoxicity

Drugs are commonly associated with acute kidney injury (AKI). The average patient demographic of today differs from that of the past. This has led to a surge in the use of more diagnostic and therapeutic procedures that carry risks to kidney function. Nephrotoxic drugs exert their detrimental effects on renal tissues via shared mechanisms. Identification of the factors that contribute to drug-induced nephrotoxicity is essential to lower the risk of kidney disease.

To prevent drug-induced kidney injury, healthcare providers need to have a comprehensive understanding of the mechanisms that underlie renal toxicity, patient-specific risk factors, drug-related risks, and proactive strategies.

Several patient-related risk factors can predispose individuals to drug-induced nephrotoxicity. These include patient age over sixty years, pre-existing renal insufficiency, volume depletion, diabetes, heart failure, and sepsis.

Drugs known for their nephrotoxic effects include Non-Steroidal Anti-Inflammatory Drugs (NSAIDs), aminoglycosides (e.g., gentamicin), vancomycin, ACE inhibitors (e.g., ramipril), diuretics (e.g., furosemide), proton pump inhibitors (e.g., omeprazole), radiocontrast agents, cyclosporine, cisplatin, methotrexate, and lithium.

Genetic factors

Once all the etiologies that cause kidney disease have been excluded, clinicians should shift focus to the family history of renal disease to identify hereditary cases. In reality, this step is conducted during the history-taking of patients. However, initial history-taking usually revolves around the risk factors and family history that increase the chances of the conditions listed above.

In recent years, research has revealed that a single-gene defect may be responsible for some kidney diseases. For instance, steroid-resistant nephrotic syndrome can cause renal disease due to podocin mutations. Consequently, it is vital to understand the most common singe-gene mutations that damage the kidneys.

Unfortunately, the management of renal disease that is caused by genetic mutations is a major challenge. Future directions may enable the development of targeted drugs that use the technology of gene therapy.

Chapter 3: Stages of Chronic Kidney Disease

What is Chronic Kidney Disease?

The two most widely accepted definitions for chronic kidney disease (CKD) were given by the Kidney Disease Outcomes Quality Initiative (KDOQI) of the National Kidney Foundation (NKF) and the Kidney Disease Improving Global Outcomes (KDIGO). KDOQI defines CKD as renal damage or a reduced estimated glomerular filtration rate of less than 60 $mL/min/1.73m^2$ for at least three months, regardless of the etiology. KDIGO defines CKD as abnormal kidney structure or function for three or more months with health consequences.

Chronic kidney disease is a continuum of metabolic and vascular abnormalities. This disease is characterized by damage to the renal parenchyma that is accompanied by irreversible sclerosis and the gradual loss of nephrons that occurs over months or years. This destruction results in a gradual loss of renal excretory, concentrating, and homeostatic functions.

The continual deterioration of individual nephrons ultimately results in the gradual deterioration of kidney function. This deterioration stems partly from cellular and molecular reactions to injury, which initially aim to restore homeostasis and compensate for the loss of nephrons but inadvertently triggers compensatory reactions that harm the remaining nephron. As nephrons are lost, the attempt of the remaining nephrons to compensate further worsens glomerular function, which causes further deterioration of kidney function.

Markers of Chronic Kidney Disease

Persistent decline of renal function, characteristic of CKD, can be distinguished by:

- Albuminuria (albumin-creatinine ratio greater than 3mg/mmol or albumin excretion more than 30mg in 24 hours).
- Abnormal urine constituents such as hematuria and red blood cell casts.
- Electrolyte derangements secondary to tubular dysfunction.
- Histological evidence of renal abnormalities.
- Radiologic evidence of structural renal abnormalities such as polycystic kidneys.

- History of renal transplant.

Factors that indicate an increased risk of advancement to more severe stages of kidney disease include the following.

- Proteinuria.
- Hematuria that originates from the kidneys.
- Decreasing glomerular filtration rate with a loss of 5 mL/min/1.73m^2 or more within a year or 10 mL/min/1.73 m^2 or more over five years.
- Diagnosis at an early age.
- Family history of renal failure.
- Resistant hypertension.

Phases of Chronic Kidney Disease

The natural history of chronic kidney disease passes through two key phases - the polyuric phase and the oliguric (or anuric) phase.

- **Polyuric phase**: In the initial stages of chronic kidney disease, the glomerular filtration rate is often sufficient for plasma urea and creatinine homeostasis. With the persistence of the insult and progressive glomerular damage, plasma levels of these key waste products begin to rise. These accumulated wastes are osmotically active. They cause left-over functional nephrons to lose fluid by osmotic diuresis, which manifests as polyuria.
- **Oliguric or anuric phase**: As more glomeruli lose the filtration function, a significant reduction in urine output and waste excretion occurs. Loss of the ability to excrete waste products causes a rapid rise in plasma urea, creatinine, and potassium levels. The accumulation of uric acid and other organic acids also becomes more apparent and results in more severe symptomatic manifestations.

Classification and Staging of Chronic Kidney Disease

The widely accepted classification of chronic kidney disease is primarily based on the estimated glomerular filtration rate (eGFR). This is because eGFR correlates closely with the risk of complications. It can also be classified based on the etiology and level of albuminuria. These classifications are highlighted in the tables below.

Table 1: Chronic Kidney Disease Classification by Estimated GFR

	eGFR (mL/min/1.73m²)	Description	Metabolic Features
G1	More than 90	Renal damage with normal or increased eGFR	Mostly normal
G2	60-89	Mildly reduced eGFR	Elevation of plasma urea, creatinine and parathyroid hormone begins
G3a	45-59	Moderately reduced eGFR	Reduction in calcium absorption Reduction in lipoprotein lipase level Reduction in erythropoietin level
G3b	30-44		
G4	15-29	Severely reduced eGFR	Derangement of lipid levels Hyperphosphatemia Metabolic acidosis Hyperkalemia Hyperuricemia
G5	Less than 15	End-stage renal failure or Renal replacement therapy (Renal transplant or Dialysis)	Severely elevated urea and creatinine

Chronic kidney disease can also be classified based on etiology thus:

Table 2: Chronic Kidney Disease Classification by Etiology

	Etiology	Examples
1	Longstanding or poorly controlled hypertension	
2	Chronic glomerulonephritis	
3	Diabetes mellitus	
4	Secondary glomerular diseases	Systemic lupus erythematosus, rheumatoid arthritis, scleroderma, granulomatosis with polyangiitis (formerly known as Wegener's granulomatosis), Goodpasture syndrome, mixed cryoglobulinemia, Hepatitides, HIV, syphilis
5	Drugs	Heroin, gold, penicillamine
6	Heredofamilial	Polycystic kidney disease, Alport syndrome, cystinosis, Fabry disease
7	Vasculitides	Polyarteritis nodosa, renal vein thrombosis, renal artery stenosis
8	Tubulointerstitial disease	Chronic hypercalcemia, multiple myeloma, cast nephropathies
9	Obstructive uropathy	Benign prostatic enlargement, prostate cancer, retroperitoneal fibrosis

Using the eGFR alone may not be sufficient for diagnosis of CKD in the early stages of CKD because the eGFR may be normal or borderline. NICE suggests clinicians use the urine Albumin-Creatinine ratio (ACR) and urine albumin excretion in such cases.

Table 3: CKD Classification by ACR and Albumin Excretion

Stage	ACR (mg/mmol)	Albumin Excretion (mg/24hr)
A1	Less than 3	Less than 30
A2	3-30	30-300
A3	Greater than 30	Greater than 300

Both eGFR and albumin excretion rates can be combined to classify chronic kidney disease in order to prognosticate and determine the best management plan for the patient. For example,

- A patient with an eGFR of 25 ml/min/1.73 m2 and an ACR of 15 mg/mmol has CKD G4A2.
- A patient with an eGFR of 50 ml/min/1.73 m2 and an ACR of 35 mg/mmol has CKD G3aA3.

It is important to note that a higher ACR is associated with an increased risk of adverse outcomes. Also, a lower eGFR is linked with more adverse outcomes. Simultaneously elevated ACR and reduced eGFR values multiply the risk of adverse outcomes.

Stage 1 Chronic Kidney Disease

Stage 1 or G1 chronic kidney disease is characterized by renal damage with a normal or elevated estimated glomerular filtration rate, usually above 90 mL/min/1.73 m^2. It is associated with an increased risk of cardiovascular diseases. Hypertension and hematuria of renal origin can also be seen in some cases. Most patients with stage 1 chronic kidney disease are usually asymptomatic. However, there may be clinical features and metabolic findings, as highlighted below.

- **Proteinuria**: Protein in the urine is often the first evidence of destruction of the glomerular basement membrane. Proteinuria presents as the frothiness of urine. Dipstick may show a trace to mild proteinuria.

- **Metabolic derangements**: Laboratory tests may reveal abnormally elevated urea and creatinine or decreased glomerular filtration rate. Other electrolyte derangements may include hyperkalemia and abnormalities in calcium and phosphate metabolism.

The primary focus in the management goal of stage 1 chronic kidney disease is to slow the progression of kidney damage and reduce risk factors for further kidney impairment.

Stage 2 Chronic Kidney Disease

Stage 2 or G2 chronic kidney disease represents a mild reduction of renal functions. The estimated glomerular filtration rate is usually between 60-89 mL/min/1.73 m^2. Like stage 1, patients with stage 2 chronic kidney disease are usually asymptomatic. Those with overt symptoms can present with any of the following.

- **Proteinuria** becomes more overt as the disease progresses.

- **Metabolic derangements**: Elevated creatinine levels, decreased eGFR, hyperkalemia, and abnormalities in calcium and phosphate metabolism become more evident as compared to stage 1.

- **Mild anemia**: Normal hematocrit ranges between 12-16 g/dL for adult females and 14-16g/dL for adult males. Hematocrit between 10g/dL and the lower limit of normal for age and sex defines mild anemia. Patients in stage 2 may experience fatigue and mild anemia due to dysfunctional erythropoietic function. Endogenous erythropoietin is produced by the renal pericytes, which are stimulated by tissue hypoxia. Erythropoietin stimulates hematopoiesis in the bone marrow. Hematuria of renal origin may also contribute to the progression of anemia in chronic kidney disease. Anemia may manifest as fatigue, dizziness, lethargy, conjunctival pallor, and reduced capillary refill time.

- **Bone and mineral disorders**: The kidney is responsible for 1-alpha hydroxylation of vitamin D. Vitamin D is essential to calcium absorption from the renal tubules and gastrointestinal tract. Early signs of bone and mineral metabolism disturbances may manifest as low levels of serum vitamin D. This can cause hypocalcemia and its accompanying clinical sequelae.

Stage 3 Chronic Kidney Disease

Stage 3 or G3 CKD represents a moderate reduction of renal function, with an estimated glomerular filtration rate ranging between 30-59 $mL/min/1.73m^2$. In addition to the features seen in the earlier stages, patients with stage 3 chronic kidney disease can present with the signs and symptoms discussed below.

- **Generalized body swelling**: The disease-mediated damage to the glomerular basement membrane causes a net protein loss. This protein loss reduces intravascular oncotic pressure and causes transudation of fluid into interstitial spaces. Accumulation of fluid in body tissues often initially manifests as early morning facial puffiness that regresses as the day goes by. With time, it becomes more generalized and persistent. Generalized edema is also known as anasarca.

- **Pruritus and skin changes**: Pruritus and skin discoloration may occur as waste products, especially uric acid, build up in the blood and become deposited in the subcutaneous tissue.

- **Oliguria or anuria**: Oliguria is defined as a urinary output of less than 400mL in 24 hours or less than 20mL per hour.

- **Anorexia and weight loss**: Reduction in appetite and urinary loss of essential body proteins in patients results in unintentional weight loss.

- **Weight gain**: Fluid accumulation in extravascular space can cause chronic kidney disease patients to gain weight. This weight is usually rapidly lost after hospitalization and commencement of treatment.

- **Urinary symptoms** like oliguria, increased frequency of daytime urination, nocturia, and frothiness of urine can occur at this stage.

Other clinical features like hyperphosphatemia, reduced vitamin D levels, anemia, and electrolyte derangements worsen at this stage. Calcium and phosphate metabolism abnormalities may cause bone pain and pathologic fractures. Dysregulation of sodium homeostasis can cause either hyponatremia or hypernatremia, with associated clinical manifestations. The risk of the occurrence of adverse cardiovascular events and associated complications is elevated in stage 3 chronic kidney diseases. Management and treatment of stage 3 chronic kidney disease is essential; the focus should be on actions that slow disease progression, manage symptoms, and address complications.

Stage 4 Chronic Kidney Disease

G4 or stage 4 chronic kidney disease (CKD) represents a severe reduction in renal function, with a glomerular filtration rate (GFR) between 15-29 mL/min/1.73m^2. Clinical features and metabolic findings in stage 4 CKD may include the following.

- **Difficulty breathing**: Fluid accumulation in the pulmonary interstitium presents as difficulty breathing, fine crackles, and orthopnea.
- **Pericarditis and pericardial effusion** can also manifest as transudation if fluid worsens.
- **Features of severe uremia**: Inadequate urea excretion leads to urea accumulation in the blood. Uremia can present as nausea, vomiting, and intractable hiccups. Cognitive impairment and difficulty with concentration may occur due to uremic encephalopathy.
- **Metabolic acidosis**: Normal body pH ranges between 7.35 and 7.45. Reduced excretion of organic acids like uric acid causes them to accumulate in the blood. Patients with metabolic acidosis can present with symptoms such as acute confusional state, fatigue, tachycardia, and shortness of breath. Dyspnea is usually due to hyperventilation caused by respiratory compensation of the metabolic problem.
- **Coagulation disorders**: Increased risk of coagulation due to loss of antithrombotic factors like antithrombin III in the urine. Loss of coagulation factors can also predispose patients with advanced chronic kidney disease to excessive bleeding.
- **Infections**: Increased susceptibility to infection due to loss of complement proteins in the urine.
- **Neurologic problems**: Polyneuropathy, autonomic dysfunction, and nerve compression can occur secondary to beta-2 macroglobulin-related amyloidosis.
- **Hypertension**: Hypertension at this stage may be difficult to control, and its effects on the cardiovascular system usually become more pronounced.
- **Increased risk of cardiovascular damage:** At this stage, the risk of an adverse cardiovascular event such as heart attack or stroke becomes significantly elevated. Cardiovascular complications are acknowledged as the primary cause of

death in individuals with end-stage renal disease (ESRD). This accounts for over 50% of fatalities during the first year of dialysis.

- **Risk of kidney failure** (end-stage renal disease, ESRD), which may necessitate dialysis or kidney transplantation.

Managing stage 4 CKD is critical and focuses on symptom relief, complication management, and preparations for possible renal replacement therapy such as dialysis and renal transplantation. Patients will need to be monitored closely and provided individualized treatment plans to maintain the best possible quality of life.

Stage 5 Chronic Kidney Disease

Stage 5 or G5 chronic kidney disease, often called end-stage renal disease (ESRD), is characterized by an estimated glomerular filtration rate below 15 mL/min/1.73m^2, indicating a critical and severe loss of kidney function. This indicates a critical and severe loss of kidney function. Patients with stage 5 chronic kidney disease usually require either hemodialysis, peritoneal dialysis, or a renal transplant to improve their chances of survival. Managing ESRD is essential for maintenance of life, and patients with stage 5 CKD often require comprehensive care from nephrologists and other healthcare providers. They may also be considered for kidney transplantation, which offers the potential for a better quality of life compared to long-term dialysis.

Chapter 4: AKI vs CKD

Acute Kidney Injury

There has been a recent shift in terminology from acute renal failure to the term acute kidney injury (AKI). AKI is a complex clinical disorder associated with significant morbidity and mortality. Despite recent technological strides in renal replacement therapy, AKI remains associated with unfavorable outcomes.

AKI is characterized by a sudden but often reversible decline in the kidneys' ability to filter and excrete waste products. It is often coupled with a reduction in urine output, which usually occurs over a period of hours to days.

Over the years, different criteria have been used to define AKI. They include risk, injury, failure, loss, end-stage kidney disease (RIFLE) criteria, Acute Kidney Injury Network (AKIN) criteria, and the Kidney Disease Improving Global Outcomes (KDIGO) criteria. The KDIGO criteria are the latest (2012) and most commonly used.

In the KDIGO clinical practice guidelines, AKI is defined as any of the following:

- An increase in serum creatinine by ≥0.3 mg/dL (26.5 umol/L) within forty-eight hours.
- An increase in serum creatinine to ≥1.5 times baseline, which is known to have occurred within the last seven days.
- A urine volume <0.5mL/kg/hr for six hours.

The occurrence of AKI varies based on the specific characteristics of the patient population, the criteria used in the definition (AKIN, RIFLE, KDIGO), and the timing of its diagnosis. Its incidence has increased in recent years due to several factors, which include improved diagnostic methods, an aging population, an increased number of underlying comorbidities, the increased use of nephrotoxic drugs, and more frequent invasive procedures. AKI affects about ten to fifteen percent of hospitalized patients and up to fifty percent of critically ill patients in the intensive care unit (ICU).

In the immediate term, AKI results in prolonged hospital stays, elevated healthcare expenses, and higher mortality rates in hospitals. In the long term, AKI has been linked with increased risks of cardiovascular incidents, progression toward CKD, and elevated mortality over an extended period. Prevention, early detection, and tailored management of AKI are essential.

Causes of AKI

AKI stems from various underlying factors, which can be categorized into three primary groups.

Prerenal AKI makes up approximately sixty percent of cases. It arises due to the kidneys' adaptive response to reduced blood flow without significant structural impairment. Intrarenal AKI accounts for about forty percent of AKI cases. It arises as a result of direct structural damage to renal tissue. Postrenal AKI (five to ten percent) occurs due to urinary tract obstructions.

AKI usually has more than one cause. It is important to grasp these distinct categories in order to understand the wide range of etiologies that can contribute to AKI.

- Prerenal AKI — The kidneys' maintenance of a normal glomerular filtration rate (GFR) depends on adequate renal perfusion. Renal hypoperfusion, either from generalized tissue hypoperfusion or selective renal ischemia, plays an important role in the etiopathogenesis of prerenal AKI. Many factors have been identified in the development of prerenal AKI. These pathways are associated with various conditions that can result in this type of kidney injury. They include:
    - Volume depletion — This can be caused by bleeding, inadequate fluid intake, fluid loss (vomiting and diarrhea), fluid shift and third space losses (pancreatitis, burns, and peritonitis), renal losses (over diuresis), and skin or respiratory losses.
    - Impaired cardiopulmonary function — This can be caused by congestive cardiac failure, cardiac tamponade, or pulmonary thromboembolism.
    - Decreased vascular resistance — This can be caused by sepsis, hepato-renal syndrome, systemic vasodilation, neurogenic shock, and anaphylaxis.
    - Intrarenal hemodynamic changes — Possible causes include the use of medications such as non-steroidal anti-inflammatory drugs (NSAIDs) like ibuprofen, Renin-Angiotensin System blockers like angiotensin-converting enzyme inhibitors (ACEIs) and angiotensin II receptor blockers (ARBs), and hypercalcemia.

- Intrarenal AKI — The causes of intrarenal AKI can be categorized based on which specific component of the kidney is affected. These components include the glomeruli, interstitial tissue, tubules, and vascular structures. This classification helps to narrow down the underlying factors that contribute to renal damage. Several conditions can damage different components of the kidney. They include:
  - Glomerular damage — This is commonly caused by acute glomerulonephritis, vasculitis, malignant hypertension, and thrombotic microangiopathies.
  - Interstitial damage — This is commonly caused by infections, which may be bacterial or viral, and medications such as antibiotics and NSAIDs.
  - Tubular damage — This is commonly caused by renal ischemia, nephrotoxins, tumor lysis syndrome, myoglobin, hemoglobin, and medications such as contrast agents.
  - Vascular damage — This is commonly caused by atheroembolism, renal artery or vein thrombosis, and vasculitis such as polyarteritis nodosa.
- Postrenal AKI — Anatomic obstruction of the urinary system at any level results in a buildup of intraluminal pressure, which can result in AKI. This can occur as a result of intrarenal or extrarenal obstruction. Causes include:
  - Intrarenal obstruction is mainly caused by nephrolithiasis, blood clots, and papillary necrosis.
  - Extrarenal obstruction can be caused by ureterolithiasis, benign prostate hyperplasia, acute neurogenic bladder, cancers (of the bladder, cervix, rectum, and prostate), urethral strictures, improperly placed catheters, retroperitoneal tumors, or fibrosis.

Characteristics of AKI

The following characteristics are observed in AKI:

- Sudden onset — As suggested, sudden onset AKI typically develops within a short period, ranging from a few hours to days.
- Change in urine production — One of the key characteristics of AKI is a noticeable change in urine production. This could present as a complete absence of urine production (anuria), a reduction in urine production (oliguria), or an increase in urine production (polyuria).
- Reversible nature — Prompt diagnosis and appropriate treatment can reverse many cases of AKI. The importance of early detection and proper management cannot be overemphasized.

- Fluid retention and edema — Due to the decline in the kidneys' function, the body retains fluid, which results in fluid accumulation (edema) in the legs, ankles, abdomen, and face.
- Azotemia and electrolyte imbalance — Azotemia is a biochemical abnormality marked by the buildup of blood urea nitrogen, creatinine, and other secondary waste products within the body. It occurs as a result of the kidney's failure to filter and excrete such waste products adequately. AKI can also result in biochemical disturbances in electrolyte balance, which can cause hyperkalemia (elevated potassium levels), hyperphosphatemia (elevated phosphate levels), and metabolic acidosis (low pH levels in the blood).

The awareness and understanding of these characteristics are essential for prompt recognition, diagnosis, and management of AKI, which significantly improves outcomes for affected patients.

Treatment Strategy for AKI

- **General measures regardless of cause:**
    - Avoid medications that could impede renal blood flow (e.g., NSAIDS). Exercise caution when using medications that have nephrotoxic properties (e.g., aminoglycosides and contrast agents and dyes).
    - Individualize patient management and tailor medication dosages to align with the patient's level of renal function.
    - Address any fluid imbalances promptly. For patients with volume depletion, intravenous fluids (IVFs) can be administered. Many patients with AKI are volume-overloaded, particularly those with oliguria or anuria. In such cases, diuretic therapy might be necessary. The goal is to find a balance between correcting volume deficit and avoiding volume overload while a steady and appropriate urine output is ensured. Daily weight measurements should be used, and a strict input and output chart should be kept.
    - When addressing fluid imbalance, it is important to consider the patient's cardiac history. Do not give excess IVF to a patient with congestive cardiac failure.
    - Address any existing electrolyte imbalance promptly. For example, correct hyperkalemia when potassium levels exceed 6.5 mmol/L to prevent cardiac arrhythmias.

- Severe acidosis can be corrected with sodium bicarbonate if the patient's volume status allows it.
- Maintain an optimal cardiac output. Aim for a blood pressure range of approximately 120 to 140 over eighty to ninety mmHg.
- Screen for intercurrent infections and treat them if present.
- Consider the initiation of dialysis in cases of symptomatic uremia, intractable acidemia, hyperkalemia, or if volume overload develops.

These general measures serve as a foundation for the treatment of AKI and set the stage for management, which addresses the likely cause of AKI.

- **General measures specific to prerenal causes:**
    - Address the root cause responsible for the prerenal AKI, e.g., hypovolemic or cardiogenic shock.
    - Administer fluids to maintain euvolemia and restore blood pressure. This should be avoided in patients with ascites or edema.
    - Remove agents that may worsen the condition, e.g., NSAIDs and ACEIs.
    - If the condition worsens and the patient becomes unstable, it may be necessary to consider intravascular volume monitoring and assessment. This can be done using a pulmonary artery catheter (Swan-Ganz catheter).
- **General measures specific to renal causes:**
    - If a renal cause, e.g., acute tubular necrosis, is suspected, the approach shifts toward the administration of supportive care while the renal function recovers.
    - During this period, identify and remove the root cause of the AKI or any agents that may contribute to the condition.
    - In patients with oliguria or anuria, a trial of furosemide may be beneficial. This diuretic can enhance urine flow, which may improve fluid balance.
- **General measures specific to postrenal causes:**
    - Insert a bladder catheter to alleviate pressure on the urinary tract.
    - Seek expert opinion from a urology specialist.
    - There may be post-obstructive diuresis and a rapid increase in urine output following relief of obstruction. This may require IVF replacement.
    - Note that the specific treatment approach will vary based on the underlying cause of the AKI, the severity, and the patient's medical history.

Prognosis for AKI

Many patients recover from AKI following supportive care. However, the prognosis of AKI is dependent on the etiology of the AKI and the presence or absence of any preexisting kidney disease or diminished GFR.

In most cases of prerenal AKI, timely intervention and correction of the root cause result in a complete recovery. However, if the underlying etiology persists, it could potentially lead to acute tubular necrosis, in which the damage may not be entirely reversible.

Isolated episodes of AKI may completely or partially resolve, but repeated occurrences can result in a cumulative and gradual decline in renal function.

In clinical settings, the in-hospital mortality rate for AKI is about forty to fifty percent, and in ICUs, it is over fifty percent.

Other prognostic factors that are considered in patients with AKI include age, illness duration, fluid balance, use of diuretics, urine output, hypotension, need for inotropic support, sepsis, multi-organ involvement, and the number of transfusions given. These factors should be collectively considered as the prognosis is assessed and individualized treatment plans are created.

Chronic Kidney Disease

CKD has emerged as a significant contributor to global morbidity and mortality rates. It is part of a group of noncommunicable diseases that have seen a rise in related fatalities in the last twenty years. This highlights the urgent need for increased focus, prevention, and effective management of CKD on a global scale.

CKD signifies an ongoing decline in kidney function that typically progresses gradually over a period of years. It is defined as a persistent abnormality in kidney structure or function lasting for more than three months. It is identified by a GFR of less than 60mL/min/ 1.73 m^2, albuminuria of at least 30 mg per twenty-four hours, or markers of kidney damage (e.g., hematuria or structural abnormalities such as polycystic or dysplastic kidneys) that persist more than three months. It is usually grouped into stages based on the estimated GFR and the presence of kidney damage. These stages range from stage one (mild kidney damage with normal or high estimated GFR) to stage five (severe kidney damage with very low estimated GFR).

CKD is underdiagnosed and affects more than ten percent of the global population, which is equivalent to over 800 million individuals. The occurrence of CKD has been rising globally, and experts predict that it will become the fifth most prevalent chronic medical condition by 2040. Its prevalence is higher in elderly populations, women, and specific racial groups. Additionally, CKD has a higher risk of occurrence in those suffering from hypertension, vascular disease, and diabetes. CKD presents a particular challenge in low- and middle-income countries, which face significant challenges in dealing with its adverse consequences.

Causes of CKD

The two most common causes of CKD globally are diabetes mellitus (twenty to forty percent of cases) and hypertension (five to twenty percent of cases).

Other causes of CKD include:

- Glomerular diseases, e.g., chronic glomerulonephritis, which accounts for ten to twenty percent of cases.
- Interstitial diseases, e.g., interstitial nephritis.
- Renovascular diseases, e.g., atheromatous narrowing of these vessels.
- Systemic inflammatory diseases, e.g., vasculitis and systemic lupus erythematosus.
- Congenital or inherited diseases, e.g., Alport syndrome and polycystic kidney disease.
- HIV-associated nephropathy.
- Sickle cell trait and genetic polymorphisms of the APOL-1 gene are associated with an increased risk of developing CKD in people of African ancestry.
- Any cause of AKI can advance to CKD if prolonged or if treatment is delayed.

Characteristics of CKD

The following are common characteristics unique to CKD:

- Reduced kidney function — In CKD, the kidneys struggle to filter waste and other substances from the blood. The resultant effect is the buildup of waste products in the body.
- Kidney damage — CKD is often associated with structural damage to the kidneys, which may result from one of several causes, e.g., diabetes mellitus, hypertension, or glomerulonephritis.
- Bilateral small or echogenic kidneys on ultrasound are common findings in advanced disease.
- Hypertension — The kidneys play a vital role in blood pressure control, so hypertension tends to develop as function declines. Hypertension is both a cause and a consequence of CKD.
- Anemia — Decreased production of the hormone responsible for stimulating red cell production (erythropoietin) causes anemia in patients with CKD.
- Fluid and electrolyte imbalance — As CKD progresses, the kidneys have difficulty regulating the body's acid-base balance, body fluids, and minerals (e.g., sodium and potassium). This results in edema and other complications, such as cardiac arrhythmias.
- Mineral and bone disorders — CKD can disrupt the balance of minerals (e.g., calcium and phosphate) in the body, which can create bone problems and increased risk of fractures.
- Uremic symptoms — In advanced stages of CKD, affected individuals may experience fatigue, gastrointestinal symptoms (such as nausea, vomiting, and anorexia), and neurological symptoms (such as memory impairment, confusion, peripheral neuropathy, and seizure).
- Bleeding secondary to platelet dysfunction.
- Immunosuppression — Uremia inhibits both cellular and humoral immunity.

Treatment Strategies for CKD

The following are treatment strategies used in the management of CKD:

- Slow down CKD progression — The root cause must first be addressed. Early detection and intense management of diabetes are important. Control of blood pressure is essential. For patients with proteinuria, medications that target the renin-angiotensin-aldosterone system (ACEIs or ARBs) are beneficial because of their blood pressure reduction, anti-inflammatory, and anti-fibrotic effects. Obese patients should be encouraged to lose weight. Smoking cessation has been associated with slower rates of progression. Patients should avoid factors that worsen kidney damage, like NSAID use. In cases of CKD with metabolic acidosis, it may be necessary to correct the acid-base balance to slow disease progression. Recent trials show sodium-glucose cotransporter-2 inhibitors, e.g., empagliflozin, can slow CKD progression even in those without diabetes or significant proteinuria.

- Dietary management — Patients with CKD will benefit from personalized dietary guidance provided by a renal nutritionist. Tailored recommendations concerning protein, salt, water, potassium, and phosphorus intake are important in slowing CKD progression and managing its associated complications.
- Medication management — The dosages of medications eliminated by the kidneys should be adjusted based on GFR. Medications that contain magnesium and phosphorus (like laxatives, antacids, and cathartics) should be avoided. Drugs with potential nephrotoxicity (like NSAIDS and intravenous contrast) should be avoided. Use of proton pump inhibitors should be employed only when necessary. For CKD patients with diabetes mellitus, a reduction in oral hypoglycemic and insulin doses should be considered as they increase the risk of hypoglycemia due to decreased renal elimination.
- Cardiovascular risk reduction — Lipid-lowering drugs (e.g., atorvastatin) benefit CKD patients as they reduce cardiovascular risk. Similarly, antiplatelet medications help in secondary prevention of cardiovascular risk.
- Anemia should be treated with erythropoietin, which is normally secreted by the kidneys.
- Pruritus should be treated with capsaicin cream or cholestyramine and ultraviolet light.
- Treatment of End Stage Kidney Disease (ESKD) — Preparation for ESKD requires a team approach that involves dieticians, social workers, primary care clinicians, and nephrologists. Whenever GFR falls to 5–10 mL/min/1.73m2, renal replacement therapy in the form of hemodialysis, peritoneal dialysis, or kidney transplantation becomes necessary. For patients with CKD, referral to a nephrologist is beneficial and should occur in late stage three or when GFR begins to decline significantly. For elderly patients or those with multiple comorbidities, dialysis may not prolong life, and the option of palliative care should be discussed with the patient and family. For healthy patients, kidney transplantation should be considered before initiating dialysis.

Prognosis for CKD

The prognosis of CKD depends on several factors, which include:

- Stage — In its early stages (one through three), lifestyle adjustments and proper management may slow or halt the progression of the disease. However, the prognosis is generally worse for patients in advanced stages (four and five).
- Root cause — The etiology responsible for CKD also influences its prognosis. CKD caused by diabetes mellitus and hypertension tend to progress and thus have a poorer prognosis.
- General patient health — The presence or absence of coexisting morbidities (such as diabetes mellitus) may influence the prognosis of CKD. Proper management of these morbidities is essential to slow or halt disease progression and thus improve prognosis.
- Age — Older patients may face more challenges in the management of CKD, which may worsen their prognosis.
- Complications — CKD patients with complications (e.g., anemia, cardiovascular disorders, and fluid and electrolyte disorders) tend to have poor prognoses and require close monitoring and management.
- Proteinuria — Leakage of excess protein in urine is a marker of kidney damage that signifies disease progression and is usually associated with poor prognoses.

Differentiating Between AKI and CKD

Factors that favor AKI	Factors that favor CKD
Sudden onset with an abrupt decline in renal function that occurs within hours to days.	Gradual onset over an extended period (months to years).
Potentially reversible.	Usually irreversible.
Caused by acute events, e.g., hypovolemia.	Caused by a prolonged, ongoing insult from diseases like diabetes and hypertension.
Symptoms develop suddenly.	Early stages are usually asymptomatic, and symptoms develop at advanced stages.
Oliguria/anuria is a common occurrence, depending on severity.	Urine output is usually normal or increased and only reduces in advanced stages.
Rapid development of azotemia.	Only develops much later at advanced stages of the disease.
Treatment is aimed at cure and reversal.	Treatment is aimed at slowing/halting disease progression.
	Small and echogenic kidney size may be seen on renal ultrasound.
	Features of chronic anemia present.
	Bone and mineral disorders may be present.
	Immunosuppression may be present.

Chapter 5: Complications of Kidney Disease

Cardiovascular Complications

Cardiovascular complications are among the leading causes of death in patients with kidney failure. They often develop in the early stages of kidney disease. Many patients struggle with cardiovascular disease even before reaching the most severe stages of kidney disease.

Hypertension

One of the most frequent side effects of chronic renal disease is secondary hypertension. It is a significant comorbidity that is connected to kidney disease. Sometimes, the severity of the glomerular disease affects the incidence and severity of hypertension. In addition to raising the risk for other cardiovascular diseases, hypertension is a complication that accelerates the rate of glomerular filtration decrease. Higher systemic pressure lowers the number of kidney nephrons which decreases the glomerular filtration rate (GFR), a measure of how effective the kidney filters toxins and metabolic products.

Development of secondary hypertension

Development of hypertension in kidney disease is a complex process that involves many factors. Some of these mechanisms include:

- Salt retention and water volume expansion.
- Sympathetic nervous system hyperactivity.
- Endothelial dysfunction.
- Upregulated renin angiotensin aldosterone system (RAAS).
- Oxidative stress.
- Vascular remodeling.

Sodium retention

Kidney disease is associated with retention of sodium due to impaired excretory functions. This retention is further influenced by aldosterone which promotes its reabsorption in the collecting tubules of the kidneys. Sodium is an osmotically active substance. It draws water along with it during reabsorption. With impaired excretory functions and the upregulated RAAS system found in kidney disease, high levels of sodium are retained along with water that causes an extracellular volume fluid expansion. This can result in fluid overload with time.

In normal circumstances the fluid overload stimulates the production of defense factors. However, the presence of kidney disease means the defense systems are overwhelmed and have no impact. The above mentioned mechanism is volume dependent. Volume independent mechanisms increase the inability of the vessels to relax and contract easily. This results in increased sympathetic outflow because of the high levels of sodium that have been retained. Normally the arterioles in the glomeruli reflexively modify their diameter in response to elevated blood pressure. However, their ability to contract and relax is reduced in this state which accentuates the progression of the kidney disease.

Renin angiotensin aldosterone system

Kidney disease results in a fall in perfusion which triggers the release of renin from the juxtaglomerular cells. This renin acts on angiotensinogen, which is produced by the liver, and converts it to angiotensin I. Subsequently, the enzyme known as angiotensin-converting enzyme (ACE) transforms angiotensin I into angiotensin II. This stimulates the release of aldosterone that promotes sodium reabsorption along with water to mediate adequate perfusion. Therefore, sodium and water retention persist and cause an overwhelming increase in extracellular volume expansion, venous return, and systemic blood pressure. Due to this effect, treatment becomes difficult.

Sympathetic nervous system

Under normal circumstances, the autonomic neuroregulation regulates the changes in heart rate and blood pressures. In chronic kidney disease, there is a failed balance between the sympathetic and parasympathetic systems. This dysfunction causes an overactivity of the sympathetic system, which in turn causes an increase in cardiac output and peripheral resistance. This adds to organ damage because there is vasoconstriction of the renal arteries and reduced blood flow. In turn, sodium is retained and this increases the sodium retention mechanism.

Vascular changes

Vascular changes can be structural and are characterized by vascular remodeling that promotes increased narrowing and loss of elasticity. This causes vascular resistance, endothelial dysfunction, reduced nitric oxide bioavailability and impaired endothelial signaling. Blood vessels in kidney disease are constantly exposed to many hormones, substances, and uremic toxins that result in these vascular changes and dysfunction. Therefore, blood vessels fail to contain the high pressure.

Heart failure

Hypertension that develops secondary to chronic kidney disease is a risk factor for heart failure. This is a complication through the mechanisms of overactive renin-angiotensin-aldosterone system (RAAS), sodium and water retention, and stiff and calcified blood vessels and heart valves. Anemia is another notable risk factor for heart failure in chronic kidney disease due to the high output condition that strains the heart. Chronic kidney disease has inflammatory and stressful effects on the heart and other organs that can result in predisposition to heart failure. Drugs used in the management of chronic kidney disease can also mediate heart failure.

Coronary artery disease

Mechanisms that predispose these patients to coronary artery disease include the association of chronic kidney disease with atherosclerosis. This occurs when calcium deposits in vascular smooth muscles narrow and render them stiff. Anemia also poses a risk with its low oxygen carrying capacity. Thus, coronary artery disease may develop in the presence of these factors. Chronic kidney disease is also associated with dyslipidemias that increase chances of atherosclerosis and eventually lead to coronary artery disease.

Arrythmias

Arrythmias in kidney disease can result from a wide range of causes. The most common type in kidney disease is atrial fibrillation. An increase in left atrial volumes can cause atrial fibrillation (AF) due to left atrial dilatation and compromised conduction. High angiotensin II levels from the overactive renin-angiotensin-aldosterone system (RAAS) cause atrial fibrosis and impair conduction of electrical impulses. This results in predisposition to AF.

Electrolyte imbalances, such as potassium and calcium, can cause ectopic and re-entry electrical activity. This plays a role in the pathogenesis of atrial fibrillation (AF).

Left ventricular hypertrophy

With increased venous return from sodium and water retention as well as anemia, the left ventricle is tasked to contract this volume at high pressure out of the heart into the systemic circulation. With time, the ventricle hypertrophies.

Pericardial disease

Accumulation of toxic metabolites and nitrogenous toxins is one of the main signs of kidney disease. These substances interact with the pericardium which causes them to release inflammatory substances. The pericardium is damaged, inflamed, and fibrosed with adhesions. Effusions can occur as well.

Increased uremia can cause pericarditis. Features of uremic pericarditis include chest pain that worsens when breathing with or without a friction rub as well as PR-interval reduction and diffuse ST-segment elevation on ECG. However, the pericardial effusion can be asymptomatic and pericarditis can be seen without significant effusion.

Metabolic Complications

Bone and mineral disorders

All skeletal abnormalities and biochemical changes are covered by the term renal osteodystrophy in patients with chronic renal failure or end-stage renal disease. Important components of this disease include disturbances in serum calcium, phosphorus, PTH, and vitamin D concentrations as well as their effects on bone remodeling, mineralization, and extra skeletal calcification.

Histopathological findings of renal osteodystrophy are often used to further classify the condition into high bone turnover conditions such as osteitis fibrosa cystica and hyperparathyroidism. Low bone turnover conditions include osteomalacia.

Mineral and bone disorder changes are seen in the metabolism of calcium, phosphorus, parathyroid hormone, fibroblast growth factor 23, and vitamin D. This also includes bone diseases whether due to renal failure or not, as well as their effects. The changes can cause arterial stiffness and calcification.

Higher phosphate and blood urea concentrations cause vascular smooth muscle cells to differentiate into cell types that can produce and deposit mineralized matrix. This product causes blood vessels and vessel walls to become calcified and stiff.

Development of mineral and bone disorders

A decrease in the rate of glomerular filtration leads to a decrease in the secretion of phosphates. Accumulated phosphates stimulate an increase in the release of parathyroid hormone and the synthesis of fibroblast growth factor 23 by the osteocytes. This effect also stimulates growth of the parathyroid gland. Fibroblast growth factor 23 reduces the activity of calcitriol, which reduces intestinal phosphate absorption. Parathyroid hormone promotes calcium absorption from bone and proximal renal tubules. The regulatory effect of fibroblast growth factor 23 on calcitriol results in decreased intestinal calcium absorption and decreased calcium levels. As the disease progresses, fibroblast growth factor 23 is persistently high. Phosphate levels begin to rise and cause secondary hyperparathyroidism. Consequences of secondary hyperparathyroidism include:

- Increased osteoclastic activity.
- Bone marrow fibrosis and cyst formation.
- Manifestations of biochemical changes such as elevated parathyroid hormone, hypocalcemia, hyperphosphatemia.
- Elevated serum alkaline phosphatase.

Parathyroid hyperplasia with tertiary hyperparathyroidism develops as parathyroid hormone is released regardless of calcium levels or other moderators. This can lead to hypercalcemia due to rapid bone turnover.

Low turnover bone disease is seen in states with reduced bone volume, excessive suppression of PTH production, or chronic inflammation. This is known as adynamic bone disease. Its complications consist of increased susceptibility to fractures, bone pain, and association with increased vascular and cardiac calcification.

Anemia

Anemia is a frequent complication of kidney disease and is often described as normochromic and normocytic. It contributes to non-specific types of symptoms in these patients. Clinical manifestations of anemia include fatigue, diminished exercise tolerance, angina, decreased cognition and mental acuity, heart failure, and impaired host defense against infection.

The primary cause is the inability of the diseased kidneys to produce erythropoietin, which is required for hematopoiesis in the bone marrow.

Other notable causes of anemia in chronic kidney disease include the following:

- Toxic effects of uremia on marrow precursor cells or fibrosis secondary to hyperparathyroidism.
- Reduced red cell survival in uremia.
- Hemodialysis may cause a degree of hemolysis.
- Blood loss due to capillary fragility and poor platelet function.
- Reduced intake, absorption and utilization of dietary iron, vitamin B12, or folate.
- Drugs such as ACE inhibitors that may interfere with the control of endogenous erythropoietin release.

Anemia in chronic kidney disease is associated with adverse pathophysiological consequences that vary from decreased tissue oxygen delivery and utilization to increased cardiac output, ventricular dilation, and ventricular hypertrophy.

Most chronic kidney disease patients may require iron supplements. Once the deficiency of iron and anemia is corrected, recombinant erythropoietin can be given. This is more effective in correcting and improving anemia and symptoms in chronic kidney disease.

Fluid, Electrolyte, and Acid-Base Imbalances

Sodium balance

Kidney disease disrupts the balance between renal excretion of sodium and intake. This causes dietary sodium intake to exceed the excretion rate and expansion of the extracellular volume. The increase in extracellular fluid volume contributes to the hypertension seen in kidney disease patients. To curb this, the patient's water intake shouldn't exceed the capacity of renal clearance. Extracellular fluid volume expansion under normal renal clearance will be isotonic and the patient will have normal plasma sodium concentration. Patients with an increased extracellular fluid volume (with peripheral edema and poorly controlled hypertension) can benefit from dietary salt restriction and thiazide diuretics. Hyponatremia is rare in these patients. However, water restriction usually resolves it.

The manifestation of diuretic resistance with intractable hypertension and edam is a sign to begin dialysis. Gastrointestinal loss of water may be difficult to correct in these patients because of the inability of the kidneys to adequately reclaim filtered sodium. Volume depletion can exacerbate kidney function and cause pre-renal factors that trigger acute deterioration in chronic kidney disease.

Potassium homeostasis

Even in kidney disease, the body strives to maintain potassium levels that are within the normal range. Potassium is controlled by aldosterone-dependent secretion in the distal nephron and augmented potassium excretion in the GI tract. Failure of these two homeostatic responses may precipitate hyperkaliemia. Though rare, hyperkaliemia can be seen in patients with increased dietary potassium intake, hemolysis, hemorrhage, transfusion of stored red blood cells, and metabolic acidosis which causes an extracellular shift in potassium. It can also occur due to drugs such as renin-angiotensin inhibitors that can inhibit renal excretion of potassium.

Hypokalemia is uncommon but it may develop in patients with gastrointestinal loss of potassium.

Metabolic acidosis

In kidney disease, there is a decreased capacity to excrete organic acids. This may lead to an anion-gap metabolic acidosis. Though these patients are able to acidify the urine, they still can't produce enough ammonia. This impairs the quantity of protons excreted. Hyperkalemia further depresses the production of ammonia, which can result in a combination of hyperchloremic-hyperkalemic metabolic acidosis. Metabolic acidosis is mild in most patients and can often be corrected with oral sodium bicarbonate supplementation.

Non-anion-gap renal tubular acidosis is seen in certain specific kidney conditions that disrupt regulation. These conditions include diabetic nephropathy and tubular interstitial disease. Though the acidosis may be asymptomatic, there is increased tissue catabolism associated with reduced protein synthesis. The presence of acidosis causes muscle wasting due to protein catabolism, bone loss due to bone buffering of acid, and accelerated progression of kidney disease.

Chapter 6: Diagnostic and Therapeutic Interventions

The kidney is a vital organ in the human body. It performs four main functions. First, it acts as an excretory organ and eliminates waste products and drug substances from the body. Second, it plays a regulatory role and maintains the balance of body fluids and compositions. Additionally, the kidney has a secretory function and produces hormones such as erythropoietin, renin, and prostaglandins. Lastly, it contributes to the metabolism of vitamin D and small, molecular weight proteins.

It is critical to understand these functions to measure kidney health and detect renal problems through laboratory and imaging investigations. The following section delves into the main renal assessment laboratory investigations and imaging modalities.

Laboratory Investigations

Urine Analysis

Urine analysis (U/A) is an invaluable diagnostic tool. It is a cost-effective and readily accessible renal test. U/A consists of three components: gross assessment, urine dipstick, and microscopy.

Gross Assessment

Color: Observe for gross hematuria or any color changes.

Amount: The normal amount is 800-2500ml/day. Oliguria is defined as ≤400ml/day, and anuria is ≤100ml/day.

Urine Dipstick

The urine dipstick detects various parameters including pH, specific gravity, heme, protein (albumin), glucose, ketones, leukocyte esterase, nitrite, and urobilinogen.

Heme: A positive result indicates hematuria, hemoglobinuria, or myoglobinuria.

Leukocyte esterase and nitrite: These indicate urinary tract infections.

Glucose: The presence of glucose in urine is observed in patients with diabetes mellitus and those with impaired tubular ability to absorb glucose, such as Fanconi Syndrome.

Ketones: A positive result is seen in diabetic ketoacidosis and starvation.

Protein: Normal protein loss in urine is generally <150 mg/day. Proteinuria, which is an increased level of protein in the urine, can be a sign of kidney damage.

Microscopy

RBC: RBCs in urine can originate from either the glomerulus or lower structures. Dysmorphic RBCs suggest glomerular origin. Uniform-shaped RBCs indicate lower structure origin.

WBC: An abnormal finding is ≥5WBC/HPF in males and ≥10WBC/HPF in women. It may indicate UTI, tubulointerstitial nephritis, or nephrolithiasis.

Casts: Cylindrical structures formed within kidney tubules due to protein coagulation. Different types of casts (hyaline casts, granular casts, muddy casts, WBC casts, and RBC casts) indicate different pathologies.

Blood Tests

Blood Urea Nitrogen (BUN)

Urea is a waste product produced by the liver during the urea cycle after protein breakdown. It is freely filtered by the glomerulus in the nephrons. Approximately 40-70% of the filtered urea is reabsorbed in the nephrons. The concentration of urea in the blood is known as blood urea nitrogen (BUN) and this is used to assess kidney function.

However, BUN levels do not reliably indicate glomerular filtration rate (GFR) as they can vary independently of GFR. BUN levels increase when GFR decreases, but they can also increase in cases of dehydration, catabolic state, high protein diet, and the use of certain drugs like glucocorticoids and tetracycline (TTC). On the other hand, BUN levels decrease with the presence of liver disease, malnutrition, old age, and SIADH, regardless of GFR.

Creatinine (Cr)

Creatinine is a waste product that is produced by the muscles during normal metabolism. It is primarily filtered by the kidney with minimal tubular reabsorption, and there is also some tubular secretion. Since it is produced at a relatively constant rate, it is considered the best indicator of the glomerular filtration rate (GFR).

However, there is a slight increase in tubular secretion of creatinine during dehydration. This can result in a slight overestimation of GFR. Additionally, certain factors such as ketoacidosis and drugs like cefoxitin, aspirin, cimetidine, and trimethoprim, can increase creatinine levels independently of GFR. Conversely, liver disease, cachexia, and advanced age can decrease creatinine levels regardless of GFR.

Despite these limitations, creatinine remains the most useful clinical test to assess renal function. The ratio of BUN to creatinine can be used as one parameter to distinguish the causes of renal insufficiency.

Glomerular Filtration Rate (GFR)

The glomerular filtration rate (GFR) is a reliable measure of kidney function. It is calculated as a determination of the volume of primary urine filtered by the kidneys per unit of body surface area. This standardized measurement is usually 1.73 m^2 and allows for accurate comparison across individuals. The average GFR ranges from 100 to 120 mL/min/1.73 m^2.

To directly measure GFR, substances like inulin or radiolabeled ethylenediamine-tetra-acetic acid (EDTA) can be injected and their clearance measured. These compounds are completely filtered at the glomerulus and are neither secreted nor reabsorbed by the renal tubules. Creatinine is widely used in GFR calculation because it provides a relatively accurate estimation of GFR. It is also easily measured in a routine blood test. However, it should be noted that a significant decline in renal function can occur before there is a noticeable rise in serum creatinine levels. The exact percentage of renal function loss at which serum creatinine begins to rise significantly can vary among individuals.

Clearance of Creatinine (liters/min) =GFR

$$\text{CrCl(ml/min)}=\frac{Urine\ Creatinine\ Concentration\left(\frac{\mu mol}{L}\right)*Volume(ml)}{Plasma\ creatinine\ concentration\ \left(\frac{\mu mol}{L}\right)*time(\text{min})}$$

There are special formulas used to calculate GFR using creatinine.

1. Cockcroft Gault CrCl= (140-age) * (Wt in kg) * (0.85 if female) / (72 * Cr).
2. MDRD (the Modification of Diet in Renal Disease) formula which considers age, sex, and race.
3. CKD-EPI (Chronic Kidney Disease Epidemiology Collaboration) equation which more accurately estimates the actual GFR than the MDRD eGFR in those with relatively preserved renal function.

Imaging Modalities in Renal Diseases

Ultrasound

Renal ultrasound is a valuable diagnostic tool that can be used to evaluate renal size and investigate potential obstructions or abnormalities in the urinary tract. It is also useful for detecting renal tumors, cysts, and stones.

Additionally, ultrasound can provide images of the prostate gland and bladder and assess bladder outflow obstruction. It can also reveal other abdominal, pelvic, and retroperitoneal conditions. In chronic kidney disease (CKD), ultrasound may show an increased signal in the renal cortex and a loss of distinction between the cortex and medulla. Doppler imaging can assess blood flow in both extrarenal and larger intrarenal vessels. This includes a measure of the resistivity index, which can be elevated in conditions like acute tubular necrosis and transplant rejection.

Computed Tomography Scan (CT scan)

Non-contrast computed tomography (CT) is considered the gold standard for diagnosis of nephrolithiasis and urolithiasis. It provides a clear view of the retroperitoneal anatomy and can differentiate between benign and malignant kidney lesions.

Contrast-enhanced CT is valuable for characterizing and assessing mass lesions within the kidney. Computed Tomography Urography (CTU) involves an initial non-contrast scan followed by the injection of contrast to evaluate cysts, tumors, and filling defects in the kidney. In cases of renal trauma, a triple-phase CT scan is used.

However, it is vital to evaluate a patient's' renal function before administering contrast agents. These agents can be nephrotoxic and may potentially worsen renal conditions if precautions are not taken when imaging is necessary.

Magnetic Resonance Imagining (MRI)

Magnetic resonance imaging (MRI) is a high-resolution imaging technique that effectively differentiates between cysts and solid masses in the kidneys. It is also an alternative to CT for visualizing renal vessels through magnetic resonance angiography (MRA).

MRA provides clear images of the main renal vessels, but it may not detect stenosis in smaller branch arteries. Caution must be exercised when using contrast agents during

MRI, as they can have potential nephrotoxic effects and may worsen existing renal conditions.

Kidney Biopsy

Kidney biopsy is a major procedure that can have a significant, life-saving impact on a patient and their treatment. However, it should only be performed by trained professionals as its accuracy relies heavily on the sample size and technique used.

There are only a few clear indications for kidney biopsy due to the potential complications it can cause. These include nephrotic syndrome in older children and adults, suspected systemic lupus erythematosus patients, acute nephritic syndrome, and unexplained acute kidney injury.

Before performing a renal biopsy, it is important to control blood pressure and perform a complete blood count and coagulation profile. This can decrease the risk of post-procedure bleeding.

The most common method of renal biopsy is percutaneous biopsy. This is dependent on the operator's experience and done through ultrasound guidance. However, other methods such as open renal biopsy, laparoscopic renal biopsy, and transjugular renal biopsy may be used if percutaneous biopsy is not possible.

Although kidney biopsy can be beneficial, it is not without risks. The major complication is bleeding, which can occur in 1.2% of cases. Bleeding may happen in three areas which include into the collecting system, underneath the kidney capsule, or into the perinephric space.

Patients should be closely monitored after the procedure for early bleeding detection. Post-biopsy care includes:

- Keep the patient supine for 4-6 hours.
- Monitor vital signs every 15 minutes for the first hour and every 30 minutes for the next four hours.
- Watch for flank pain and hematuria.

Routine evaluation of a percutaneous kidney biopsy involves examination of the tissue under light, immunofluorescence, and electron microscopy. The immunofluorescence examination should include evaluation of IgG, IgM, IgA, C3, C4, C1q, albumin, fibrin, and kappa and lambda immunoglobulin chains. These findings can significantly impact treatment and prognosis.

Below are histological findings of some renal pathologies.

Table 4: Histologic findings of renal pathologies

Pathology	**Features of light microscopy**	**Features of immunofluorescence microscopy**	**Features of electron microscopy**
Membranous nephropathy	- Diffuse thickening of glomerular basement membrane in all glomeruli	- IgG and C3 staining	- Sparse or no effacement of foot processes
Anti GBM disease	- Crescentic glomerulonephritis	- Linear deposition of IgG on glomerular capillaries	- No deposits
Focal segmental glomerulosclerosis	- Segmental sclerosis, hyalinization	- Negative	- Effaced podocyte foot process
Lupus nephritis	- Dependent on stage	- Full house immunofluorescence pattern - (IgG, IgM, IgA, C3, C1q)	- Thickening of the GBM, mesangial expansion, endothelial cell

			swelling, and podocyte foot process effacement

Treatment Modalities

Dialysis

Dialysis is a treatment that serves as a replacement for kidney function to remove waste from the body. It significantly increases the life expectancy of individuals with chronic kidney disease and end-stage renal disease. Dialysis does not aid in the preservation of kidney function but rather provides a substitute for the lost function during acute kidney injuries. It removes waste products and excess fluid from the blood when the kidneys are not functioning properly.

Indications to initiate patients on dialysis include but are not limited to uremic symptoms, refractory hyperkalemia, refractory acidemia, refractory fluid overload, bleeding diathesis, and a GFR of less than 10.

Renal replacement therapies come in two types: hemodialysis and peritoneal dialysis.

Hemodialysis involves the diffusion of waste materials across a partially permeable membrane. It requires three essential components:

- Dialyzer eliminates waste and retains larger molecules.
- Dialysate is a fluid that removes waste products from the blood with a specific composition of electrolytes tailored to the patient's needs.
- Dialysis machine includes a blood pump, a delivery system for dialysis solution, and monitoring devices.

Dialysis access is also critical, with an arterial and venous route through a fistula, graft, or catheter.

Hypotension is the most frequent complication of hemodialysis. It can be resolved through discontinuance of the dialysis or administration of an intravenous isotonic solution. Another common complication is nonfunctional hemodialysis access. This might necessitate the cooperation of a multidisciplinary team of interventional radiologists, vascular surgeons, and nephrologists to establish another route. Other infrequent complications include anaphylactic reactions to the dialysate, chest pain, fever, and intradialytic hypertension.

The second type of renal replacement therapy is peritoneal dialysis. This involves use of the patient's peritoneal membrane as the partially permeable membrane. While peritoneal dialysis is commonly used for chronic dialysis, it can also be used in some acute settings, although it is less commonly chosen than hemodialysis for emergent needs. The suitability of peritoneal dialysis for acute renal failure depends on the patient's clinical condition and other factors.

A sterile solution called dialysate is introduced into the peritoneal cavity through a catheter. Waste products diffuse across the membrane into the solution, which is then drained out. Peritoneal dialysis can be done at home by the patient or caregiver, and does not require a machine.

Peritoneal dialysis can be continuous ambulatory peritoneal dialysis or automated peritoneal dialysis. Continuous ambulatory peritoneal dialysis (CAPD) is a type of peritoneal dialysis that involves the continuous exchange of dialysis fluid (dialysate) into and out of the peritoneal cavity. This is done manually. Automated peritoneal dialysis (APD) uses a machine called a cycler to perform exchanges of dialysate while the patient sleeps.

The most common complication of peritoneal dialysis is peritonitis which is infection of the peritoneum. Pain with cloudy dialysate and fever are common symptoms. If suspected, it should be approached with a septic workup. This includes cell count of the peritoneal fluid with differentials, gram stain, and culture. Treatment should be started empirically as soon as possible with targeted treatment after results arrive. Staph. aureus is the most common culprit.

Other complications include non-peritonitis catheter-associated infections, electrolyte abnormalities, and hypoproteinemia.

Renal Transplantation

The method of treatment choice for end-stage renal disease is kidney transplantation. There are only a few absolute contraindications for this procedure. These are active infections, active malignancy, ongoing substance use disorder, documented drug nonadherence, untreated psychiatric illness, and treatable kidney failure. Significantly jeopardized life expectancy is a relative contraindication.

Candidates for renal transplant undergo a thorough evaluation. This includes but is not limited to documentation of the nature of renal disease and other medical comorbidities, surgical procedures, and psychiatric conditions. They also undergo a psychosocial evaluation to assess their understanding, readiness, and social support. Thorough laboratory testing for CBC, metabolic panel, coagulation studies, urinalysis, blood typing, HLA typing, screening for previous and current infections, chest x-ray, ECG, and echocardiography are among the list of investigations.

Donors can be deceased or living relatives. Living volunteer donors should undergo screening to ascertain their ability to donate. Deceased donors should be screened for infections and malignancies.

The surgery is invasive and involves placing the transplanted kidney in the extraperitoneal space in the lower abdomen, often in the iliac fossa, not the inguinal fossa. Although the peritoneal cavity is normally not entered during this procedure, the surgery itself is still considered invasive.

The transplant surgery is followed by immunosuppressive therapy. This is divided into induction therapy and maintenance.

Induction therapy is given immediately after the transplant to prevent rejection of the transplanted kidney. This usually involves a combination of medications such as antithymocyte globulin, basiliximab, or alemtuzumab. Maintenance therapy is given long-term to prevent rejection and includes medications such as calcineurin inhibitors, mycophenolate mofetil, and corticosteroids.

Regular follow-up is vital after the transplant to monitor for any complications or signs of rejection. This includes regular blood tests to monitor kidney function and medication levels, as well as imaging studies to assess the transplanted kidney.

Chapter 7: Hemodialysis

Types of Hemodialysis

Introduction

End-stage renal disease (ESRD) is a chronic illness characterized by a progressive decline in kidney function. ESRD is a glomerular filtration rate (GFR) of less than 15 mL per minute. If no intervention is made, uremia will ensue and, eventually, death. The only available cure for ESRD is renal transplant. A renal transplant has limitations due to difficulty securing a "donor kidney." Some patients may be on the waiting list for a long time.

Hemodialysis is a treatment modality available to serve as an artificial, extracorporeal kidney. It is not a cure for ESRD. The main goal of hemodialysis is to act as the kidney and provide fluid balance for patients who do not have proper kidney function. This is achieved by removing excess fluid and waste products (e.g., urea, creatinine) from the blood. This method is extracorporeal, which means that it is done outside the body through specialized equipment.

During hemodialysis, there is diffusion of molecules through a semipermeable membrane through an electrochemical concentration gradient. A concentration gradient is the difference in concentration of a solute in two areas. The higher the concentration of solute on one side, the higher the concentration gradient and the faster the diffusion rate. An electrochemical concentration gradient is the electric potential of the ions that are transferred across the semipermeable membrane. This creates both a chemical force and an electric force. These gradients affect the movement of solute across the membrane.

Hemodialysis uses counter-current exchange with the use of a dialysate. Dialysate contains a solution of pure water, some salts (e.g., sodium and bicarbonate), and electrolytes. It is also called a dialysis solution, bath, or dialysis fluid. During dialysis, the blood and dialysate flow in opposite directions. This opposite flow ensures that the concentration gradient across the semipermeable membrane remains at its highest. As a result, the efficiency of the dialysis process is significantly improved. Fluid is removed by alteration of the hydrostatic pressure of the dialysate part. This process is called ultrafiltration.

Consequently, water and solutes dissolved in it shift through the membrane along the pressure gradient. The waste products in the blood (e.g., urea, creatinine, potassium, phosphate) diffuse into the dialysate. The concentrations of sodium and chloride in the dialysate are carefully adjusted and may not always be similar to their concentrations in the patient's plasma. The composition of the dialysate is tailored to achieve the desired electrolyte balance and fluid removal for each individual patient. A high concentration of sodium bicarbonate is added to the dialysate solution to correct any acidity in the blood. Glucose may also be added if needed.

With the advent of hemodialysis, survival for people diagnosed with end-stage renal disease (ESRD) is possible. Since its discovery decades ago, different techniques have been developed for dialysis. Hemodialysis modalities can be classified based on different parameters that include:

- Classification based on the features of the dialyzer, dialysate, and blood flow.
    - Low-flux hemodialysis.
    - High-flux hemodialysis.
    - Extended hemodialysis.
    - Hemodiafiltration.

- Classification based on the location in which the procedure is carried out.
    - In-center (treatment provided within the hospital or specialized dialysis center).
    - Home (treatment is done at the home of the patient).
    - In-center self-care hemodialysis (the treatment occurs in a center, but the patient is in charge of dialysis administration).
- Classification based on the presentation of the patient.
    - Acute hemodialysis (patients who are acutely ill and require urgent dialysis due to acute or chronic renal failure).
    - Chronic hemodialysis (chronic renal failure or ESRD on continuous dialysis).
- Classification based on the number of dialysis sessions.
    - Conventional hemodialysis.
    - Daily hemodialysis:
        - Short daily hemodialysis.
        - Nocturnal hemodialysis.

Dialysis centers may provide some or even all of these different techniques for dialysis. They have protocols and guidelines for the modalities available in their center.

The management of a patient on dialysis requires a multidisciplinary team that consists of a nephrologist, nurse, nutritionist, and other condition-based support staff. This team will guide patients to determine the best modality based on their current situation. The decision to use a particular modality of dialysis (conventional or daily) depends on many factors:

- The age of the patient.
- The clinical history of the patient (this includes their clinical progression, comorbidities, and treatment received).
- The patient's body surface area.
- The presence of comorbidities such as heart failure or chronic lung disease.
- Hemodialysis access (vascular).
- The services provided by the dialysis center.
- The patient's preference for home dialysis or in-center treatment, personal beliefs, and values.
- The patient's situation in terms of renal transplantation.
- The condition of the dialysis center.

In this section, the discussion will be about the different types of hemodialysis. These types will be based on the frequency of procedures along with their advantages and disadvantages.

Conventional Hemodialysis

Conventional hemodialysis is one of the main treatment methods for treating end-stage renal disease (ESRD) patients. It is the most common dialysis modality practiced in many parts of the world. Conventional hemodialysis is a type of dialysis done about three to four times weekly. Each session can last for about three to four hours. It can take up to five hours for larger patients. It is usually done for patients who have ESRD but are stable.

The conventional hemodialysis technique operates on the concept of simple diffusion. Toxins in the blood (the region of high concentration) are removed through a filter (semipermeable membrane) into the dialysate (the region of lower concentration). The dialyzer type used is usually low-flux. A low-flux dialyzer or filter has a low permeability for water. The water is removed at a lower rate. The molecules filtered out are soluble in water and have a molecular weight of less than five hundred Daltons. Originally, acetate dialysate was the standard option in dialysis treatment. However, improvements in technology occurred, and bicarbonate dialysate became more prevalent.

Conventional hemodialysis can be done either in-center or at home up to three times a week. The patient does not get dialysis for the rest of the four days. This arrangement favors fluid accumulation between dialysis sessions (interdialytic interval). Fluid overload results in hemodynamic instability, a precursor for heightened cardiovascular morbidity and mortality.

Cardiovascular complications are among the most common causes of death associated with hemodialysis.

Advantages of Conventional Hemodialysis

- Removes excess fluid and toxins from the body, such as urea and creatinine.
- Improved survival rate in patients with ESRD.
- Correction of fluid, electrolyte, and acid-base imbalances.

Disadvantages of Conventional Hemodialysis

- Despite its contribution to improving the survival rate of ESRD patients, conventional hemodialysis has not been able to replace the normal physiology of the kidneys. Although conventional hemodialysis cannot fully replicate the functions of a healthy kidney and may perform a limited percentage of a normal kidney's function, it remains an essential and lifesaving treatment option for patients with ESRD. It provides vital functions like the removal of toxins and excess fluid, and the balancing of electrolytes. It significantly improves the quality of life in ESRD patients.
- There is an increase in blood pressure and excessive fluid accumulation in the body between two dialysis sessions (interdialytic interval). The cardiovascular system may be affected by fluid overload and high blood pressure, hence the need for proper fluid management. Before starting hemodialysis, the patient's volume status must be assessed.
- Conventional hemodialysis is associated with a high risk for cardiovascular complications caused by volume overload or hypertension.
- There is less hemodynamic stability during dialysis due to the long interdialytic gap.

- There is an increased need for medication to control blood pressure and phosphate levels.
- There is a high degree of malnutrition and increased phosphate levels in the blood (hyperphosphatemia).
- Conventional hemodialysis dramatically impacts the patient's quality of life and the need for rehabilitation.
- Higher rate of hospitalization compared to other dialysis types.
- Patients may experience dizziness or cramps during conventional hemodialysis due to the high rates of ultrafiltration or accumulated fluid in the body.

Hemodiafiltration

Over many decades, the idea of conventional hemodialysis has changed with the advancement of clinical knowledge and technology. There has been a change in the control of hemofiltration and extensive use of bicarbonate dialysate as opposed to the use of acetate dialysate that was initially used. This has led to improved blood flow during dialysis and encourages the use of synthetic high-flux dialyzers. Acetate dialysate was used previously with low blood flow rates, low-flux dialyzers, and no volume control on dialysis machines. However, with technological advancements, a new era of hemodialysis has been achieved with high-flux hemodialysis, hemofiltration, and hemodiafiltration. Hemodialysis can now be done with synthetic dialyzers.

Hemodiafiltration uses the technique of convection in addition to the diffusion principle. Convection is a process in which the solute and the solvent move across a membrane. The rate of convection depends on the characteristics of the semipermeable membrane. Hemodiafiltration has a significant advantage in the clearance of larger molecules by convection. It requires membranes with high biocompatibility, high flux, and efficiency, with close ultrafiltration control. The dialysis fluid should be highly pure. A high ultrafiltration rate of four to thirty liters is used per session.

Hemofiltration

Hemofiltration involves the use of a fluid, and is often referred to as replacement fluid. It is infused into the blood either before (pre-dilution) or after (post-dilution) it passes through the filter. This process helps to remove solutes via convection.

Short Daily Hemodialysis

This technique of hemodialysis has gained popularity over the decades. The reason is because of the frequency of dialysis sessions the patient receives. Daily dialysis comes close to normal kidney function, which is more advantageous than the conventional method. Over the years, many complications have arisen in patients undergoing conventional hemodialysis.

In short daily hemodialysis, the procedure is done for one and a half to two and a half hours over six to seven days a week. This way, the patient receives dialysis as frequently as possible to mimic the normal kidney function that filters blood twenty-four hours a day. As a result, many dialysis centers have added daily dialysis to their services.

Short daily hemodialysis has a more constant concentration of solutes. The concentrations of urea, creatinine, hydrogen ions, and potassium before dialysis are lower. As a result, ultrafiltration rates are lower. This provides better cardiovascular stability.

Advantages of Short Daily Hemodialysis

- Short daily dialysis increases the procedure frequency, which provides close to normal kidney function.
- Short daily hemodialysis has better hemodynamic stability because it decreases fluid accumulation in the body between dialysis sessions.
- Uremic toxins are filtered more effectively with the short daily hemodialysis.
- Short daily hemodialysis has a better survival rate with improved blood pressure control, less need for antihypertensive medications, better phosphate balance, better appetite, decreased rate of hospital admissions, and improved quality of life.

Disadvantages of Short Daily Hemodialysis

- There could be increased complications associated with vascular access in the short daily hemodialysis technique, such as an increased risk of thrombus formation in the fistula. However, the risk can be decreased by cannulating the fistula via the buttonhole method.
- Although short daily hemodialysis may lead to a lower hospital admission rate and a lesser need for medication, the overall cost of this modality can be higher due to the increased frequency of treatments.

Nocturnal Hemodialysis

Nocturnal dialysis is done between six to eight hours for three or more days a week at night. The procedure can be done either in the dialysis center or at home. Nocturnal hemodialysis is now practiced in many parts of the globe, although its prevalence is unknown.

Patients who opt for home nocturnal hemodialysis must be physically and mentally fit to administer the treatment at home or have a reliable care partner who can do it. Training the patient and assessing their ability to administer the hemodialysis successfully is necessary.

In-center nocturnal hemodialysis could be done for patients not qualified for hemodialysis at home. Patients who may need in-center nocturnal hemodialysis are physically unable to perform the dialysis independently, do not have a suitable care partner, or prefer to have support from nurses and other medical staff.

Advantages of Nocturnal Hemodialysis

- Home nocturnal hemodialysis allows the patient to have a flexible dialysis schedule. They have the option to have dialysis more than three times a week.
- Better cardiovascular outcomes have been noted with nocturnal dialysis. Cardiac remodeling is favorable. There is a decrease in left ventricular hypertrophy and better blood pressure control. This causes a decreased need for antihypertensive drugs.
- A better survival benefit has been reported in some observational studies.
- Long nocturnal hemodialysis has better hemodynamic stability due to a slower ultrafiltration rate during dialysis.
- The cost-effectiveness of home nocturnal hemodialysis compared to conventional in-center dialysis can vary widely depending on several factors, including the healthcare system, the specific setup and operational costs at home, and individual patient circumstances. There is less expenditure on labor (nursing staff) and less use of drugs. It is important to note that the cost of dialysis may vary across different facilities.
- Improved clearance of solute because of the regular frequency of the dialysis sessions. More phosphate can be cleared out as a result.
- Nocturnal hemodialysis helps to partially restore the melatonin rhythm with a better physiologic sleep cycle.

- There is a reduction in the need for erythropoiesis-stimulating agents and enhanced anemia management.
- Nocturnal hemodialysis may favor conception with an increased rate of improved pregnancy outcomes.

Disadvantages of Nocturnal Hemodialysis

- In home nocturnal hemodialysis, patients and their care partners must be taught how to administer the treatment at home and use the dialysis machine and other appliances.
- A physical space at home must be used during the therapy and to store the equipment and supplies.
- This modality requires the patient to be motivated to go through the treatment. It is challenging to administer treatment to oneself while living with a chronic condition. Patients and their caregivers must clearly understand the condition and treatment plan and be able to follow it.
- Home nocturnal hemodialysis needs a multidisciplinary team, such as nephrologists, nurses, nutritionists, and social workers.

Below is a summary of the different hemodialysis modalities discussed in this section and their characteristics:

Table 5: Types of Hemodialysis and Their Different Characteristics

Hemodialysis type/modality	Number of sessions per week	Duration of each session	Rate of dialysate flow (mL/min)	Rate of blood flow (mL/min)	Type of vascular access
Conventional hemodialysis	Three to four sessions	Three to five hours	500	300	All
Short daily hemodialysis	Six to seven sessions	One and a half hours to three hours	500-800	400-500	All
Nocturnal home hemodialysis	Five to seven sessions	Six to eight hours	200-300	200-350	Any suitable access, including AV fistula, AV graft, or central venous catheter, depending on patient suitability and circumstances.
Nocturnal in-center hemodialysis	Three sessions	Eight hours	500	300-400	All

It is important to note that observational studies are mainly used to investigate the risks and benefits of hemodialysis due to challenges in conducting higher-quality studies.

Chapter 8: Patient Assessment and Care Planning

Pre-dialysis Assessment

Vital Signs Assessment

The specific vitals monitored in the pre-dialysis assessment include blood pressure, temperature, pulse, and respiratory rate.

Hypertension is prevalent among chronic kidney disease patients. Hypertension is defined as an elevation of the systolic blood pressure above 140mmHg and/or diastolic blood pressure above 90mmHg on more than two occasions, measured 4-6 hours apart. Hence, blood pressure is the most common vital sign assessed in pre-dialysis. The recommended goal for high blood pressure in a CKD patient is 130/80 mmHg. A sustained elevated blood pressure further damages the kidneys and increases the need for hemodialysis.

Temperature, pulse, and respiration serve as baseline vitals pre-dialysis. Any variation requires proper investigation and management. A high temperature (>99.3 degrees Fahrenheit) may indicate an illness or vascular access infection. A rapid elevated pulse (>100 beats per minute) may indicate anemia or fluid overload, which is common in CKD. The standard pulse rate is between 60-100 bpm. An increased respiratory rate greater than 20 breaths per minute could also signify massive edema.

Weight Assessment

Dialysis patients require weight assessment before and after hemodialysis. The weight shows the level of fluid balance control by the patient. Pre-dialysis weight is a good predictor of the required ultra-filtration during dialysis. Most dialysis centers recommend a daily weight gain of around 1 pound.

Fluid Assessment

Fluid assessment occurs via a general physical examination. Predictors of fluid overload include distended neck veins, pedal and generalized edema, and increased respiratory rate.

Fluid assessment determines the needed ultrafiltration in dialysis. The goal of fluid assessment is to prevent dehydration and fluid overload. Signs of dehydration often present as sunken eyes, limited tear production, and parched lips. The oral mucosa may also appear dry, and an intense thirst may develop. The skin may lose its elasticity, known medically as "turgor," and the capillary refill time can slow. Patients may also exhibit a feeble pulse and decreased urine production.

Dialysis Prescription and Individualized Care Planning Based on the Patient's Needs and Comorbidities

The management of a patient on hemodialysis is individualized and based on the patient's diagnosis, needs, and health concerns. This is reflected in the number of times a patient undergoes hemodialysis, the number of minutes spent on each session, and the intensity of each session.

Diabetes Mellitus

Diabetic patients on hemodialysis are vulnerable and require specialized care. Individualized care plans for these patients involve self-monitoring blood glucose levels before and after dialysis. The optimal pre-dialysis blood glucose range for diabetic patients can vary, but generally, maintaining blood glucose levels below 180 mg/dl is often targeted to avoid hyperglycemia while also minimizing the risk of hypoglycemia during and after dialysis. A glycated hemoglobin value range of 6-8% is also acceptable. In addition, doctors often recommend basal-bolus insulin therapy, with a 10-15% reduction in dosage on dialysis days. Diabetic patients demand personalized dietary and nutritional assistance. Thus, proper counseling and handling of complications become vital for individuals diagnosed with diabetes mellitus.

Hypertension

Hypertension is a significant cause of death among CKD patients undergoing hemodialysis. It is a leading etiological factor for CKD. Pre and post-dialysis values of <140/90 mmHg are the recommended values for patients. Individualized care aids in reaching the desired outcome. Initially, one must restrict dietary sodium to prevent weight gain and edema.

Calcium channel blockers, ACE, and ARB blockers are essential for blood pressure control in dialysis patients who require antihypertensive therapy. Regular blood pressure monitoring and comprehensive guidance on hypertension complications are vital.

Chronic Liver Disease

Patients diagnosed with liver cirrhosis are at risk of CKD. This risk further increases the morbidity and mortality in such patients. Patients may ultimately need dialysis and personalized care. This care often encompasses routine electrolytes, urea, and creatinine checks. Regular urine examinations are vital for the early detection of any pathological alterations. In the event of spontaneous bacterial peritonitis, antibiotic therapy becomes an integral part of personalized care. Additionally, for patients suffering from hypo-albuminemia, albumin therapy can enhance their prognosis. In cases of resistant renal diseases, doctors recommend renal replacement therapy.

Heart Failure

Heart failure patients on dialysis have special individualized needs. These needs include dietary modification, which helps reduce harmful cholesterol levels. Also, regular physical exercise is essential to ensure the functional pumping of the heart. These patients require education on regular blood pressure monitoring.

Sometimes, hemodialysis can precipitate or worsen heart failure. Factors that can worsen heart failure in dialysis patients include left ventricular diastolic dysfunction, valvular heart disease, arterial stiffness, and left systolic dysfunction. An ECG and ECHO must be done before hemodialysis on “at-risk” patients.

Diabetes mellitus frequently occurs in heart failure patients. Therefore, these patients require regular checks of their blood glucose levels. In addition, lifestyle changes such as quitting smoking and reducing alcohol intake can enhance disease prognosis. Regular hospital check-ups and medication reviews remain critical. Finally, for those patients with anemia, consistent PCV evaluations are necessary to determine the need for hematinic prescriptions.

Chapter 9: Vascular Access for Hemodialysis

Overview

Hemodialysis (HD) requires access to the circulation to remove and return blood to the patient. Hemodialysis typically uses an arteriovenous fistula, arteriovenous graft, or a central venous catheter for vascular access. In the case of an arteriovenous fistula or graft, there is only one access point needed because the same site is used for both drawing blood from and returning it to the patient's circulation, not separate arterial and venous access points. With a central venous catheter, there are two lumens in the catheter, but it still constitutes a single access point.

The establishment and maintenance of vascular access in Chronic Kidney Disease (CKD) patients provides more significant challenges than acute vascular access. Adequate dialytic therapy requires reliable and long-term access to circulation, which is best achieved by constructing an endogenous arteriovenous fistula.

The attainment and maintenance of a single reliable, long-lasting dialysis access with minimal complications remain challenging. Achieving this type of access is associated with optimal patient clinical outcomes, superior quality of life, and minimal costs.

It is vital to adopt a multidisciplinary team approach in which all renal replacement therapy options are understood and considered to ensure the best possible outcome. By doing so, the patient can secure optimal access at various key stages throughout their CKD journey.

This multidisciplinary vascular access team includes the nephrologist, surgeon, endovascular interventionists, vascular access coordinator, nurse, and patient.

For individuals with end-stage renal failure, the vascular access must be reliable. About 25% of hospital hospitalizations for dialysis patients are due to access-related problems, and access failure is a substantial cause of morbidity.

Healthcare staff should be trained in patients with CKD to preserve arm veins. All individuals with renal illness should not undergo subclavian catheterization or have IV lines placed in their forearm cephalic veins. Dialysis access planning should start in CKD stage IV when education about CKD and modalities of renal replacement therapy are discussed. The rate of decline of GFR over time is usually the best predictive guide to timely referral and providing vascular access. The additives required for patient-centered access planning are:

- Timely and appropriate referral.
- Education.
- Patient history and physical examination.
- Supportive investigations.

Dialysis units should create vascular access alternatives to minimize the problems brought on by poor access. The proposed methods are:

- Maximize AVF use.
- Plan AVF formation in CKD patients as early as possible.
- Decrease the occurrence of infections and thrombosis.
- Detect access at risk for thrombosis and failure.

Arteriovenous Graft (AVG), Central Venous Catheter (CVC), and Arteriovenous Fistula (AVF) are the three vascular access methods commonly utilized for hemodialysis.

Arteriovenous Fistula (AVF)

AVF is still the best form of permanent vascular access. It is commonly made by anastomosing the cephalic vein and radial artery at the wrist, either end-to-side or side-to-side. In AVF rather than AVG, there is strong evidence for long-term patency, fewer complication rates, decreased morbidity, and increased function over time.

Consideration of access location necessitates a meticulous, systematic progression from one vascular access site to another. This process aims to conserve and utilize every available site, which prolongs the patient's lifeline in the face of end-stage renal disease. In that order, the preferred locations for AVF are radiocephalic, radiobasilic, brachiocephalic, and brachiobasilic transposition.

AVF needs to be planned at least one or two months before starting hemodialysis, a time required for the proper maturation of the fistula. A duplex ultrasound scan allows for the evaluation of the arterial and venous diameters and is the gold standard for determining the specific type and location of the fistula. AVF maturation is predicted by a vein diameter of more than 2 mm and an artery diameter of more than 1.6 mm. The timing related to the achievement of these characters ranges from one to three months.

The main advantage of an AVF is a matured, carefully cannulated, and functioning fistula that can provide reliable, long-standing access to dialysis with minimal complications. This means it provides the patient with high satisfaction and a good quality of life while remaining cost-effective.

The most common complication of AVF is maturation failure, which occurs in 20-60% of patients. Other issues include thrombosis, aneurysm development, and steal syndrome, which occurs when arterial inflow becomes restricted and flows through the fistula or graft less resistant than other distal vascular beds. In extreme circumstances, it could result in digital gangrene. The failure of AVF is usually related to stenosis of the artery or vein. Endovascular or surgical procedures can usually correct this.

Fistula infections can vary with cannulation technique. While buttonhole cannulation has been associated with an increased risk of local infections, it is not limited to exceptional circumstances only. Buttonhole technique is often used for patients who perform home hemodialysis or have difficulty with other cannulation techniques. It is a viable and regularly used method, not just limited to cases with short or limited cannulation length and large aneurysmal fistulas. Proper technique and hygiene are crucial to minimize infection risks with buttonhole cannulation.

Arteriovenous Graft (AVG)

An arteriovenous graft (AVG) utilizes a synthetic conduit interposed between an artery and a vein to connect the two vessels that are anatomically separated. The AVG has dual functionality. It allows arterial blood flow into the venous system and provides vascular access for hemodialysis.

AVG is rarely indicated as the first line of treatment and is usually the second step of treatment after an AVF is made with native vessels.

A clinical evaluation of the upper limb is necessary for proper AVG planning. Important things to consider include skin integrity and the presence of superficial veins. The presence of peripheral pulses should also be evaluated. The second step is the duplex ultrasound exam, which provides indications of upper limb artery patency and the presence of stenosis or occlusions that should be treated before restoring adequate flow.

The synthetic graft is one of the permanent vascular access. It is usually made from PTFE (polytetrafluoroethylene). The material is porous, which allows for the growth of fibroblasts and the incorporation of the graft into the subcutaneous tissues. Other synthetic and biological materials can be used for synthetic grafts. Examples of synthetic material-based grafts include PTFE variants and Dacron. Examples of biological material-based grafts include bovine heterografts, bovine mesenteric veins, human umbilical veins, and engineered human extracellular matrix compositions.

The purpose of grafts is to connect two vessels that may not otherwise be possible because of their distance. As a result, a graft can be used for almost any patient if the patient has acceptable receiving vessels. Within 3 to 4 weeks, fibrous tissue secures the graft in its subdermal tunnel and helps achieve hemostasis at needle puncture sites. PTFE can withstand numerous thrombectomies and revisions. However, these grafts are more prone to thrombosis and infection than primary AV fistulas.

The most typical method is a forearm loop that extends 10 cm down the forearm and connects the brachial artery and cephalic vein. Additionally, upper arm loop grafts, upper arm grafts, and upper thigh femoral loops are installed. Puncturing short grafts repeatedly at just a handful of places can cause them to disintegrate. In contrast, long grafts have increased pressure, reduced flow, and increased thrombosis risk.

Even though grafts have a lower early failure rate than AVFs, they can be used soon after creation. Early cannulation grafts can be used within 24 hours of creation. Standard grafts can be used 2-4 weeks after creation. As a result, arteriovenous grafts provide an acceptable alternative in patients where arteriovenous fistula is impossible.

The most common complication of grafts is the development of recurrent stenosis and thrombosis. Other disadvantages include extensive surgery, increased risk of infection, and a shorter expected life of 3 to 5 years. It is also substantially more difficult to remove and can cause skin erosions.

Central Venous Catheter (CVC)

Central venous catheters (CVCs) are a type of vascular access that can be used both for short-term and long-term hemodialysis. This method mainly applies to situations demanding urgent hemodialysis or the initiation of renal replacement therapy. It also proves useful when permanent access suffers a dysfunction or in cases where poisoning necessitates short-term hemodialysis.

The devices made of polyurethane are readily available and can be inserted into various sites of the body. Maturation time is not required, which allows immediate hemodialysis.

The internal jugular, femoral, and subclavian veins are potential sites for insertion. The possibility of subclavian stenosis, which could jeopardize future fistulas, should prevent any patients needing permanent access from undergoing the subclavian approach. The femoral route should only be used in bedridden or immobile patients. It can also be helpful in patients who cannot lie flat for line insertion. However, it has the highest infection risk. Bedside ultrasound can accurately locate the target vein and provide information about venous pressure and the presence of intravascular thrombus.

This temporary vascular access can be tunneled or non-tunneled. Non-tunneled access can be inserted at the bedside under ultrasound control. It should be placed immediately before use and have its position confirmed by radiography.

Infection risks are higher with non-cuffed catheters, especially if left in place for more than five days. The duration for which femoral and internal jugular catheters are left in place can vary based on clinical need and individual patient factors. Femoral catheters can be used for longer than 1-3 days if necessary, especially in certain clinical situations like critical illness.

The cuffed and tunneled type is inserted within the subcutaneous tissue under ultrasonographic and fluoroscopic guidance to reach the target vein.

Regardless of the location, a modified Seldinger approach is used to insert a central venous catheter. It should be done under ultrasound guidance to visualize the vein and with an assistant under fully sterile conditions. Ultrasound guidance can reduce complications, and each patient must be individually assessed for factors that might improve or worsen any location. These conditions include obesity, infections, and chronic obstructive pulmonary disease.

The advantages of a central venous catheter include ease of insertion, low cost, ease of change, and immediate usability. The disadvantages include infection, venous stenosis, venous thrombosis, local complications, short life, and easy dislodgment.

Nursing Care for Vascular Access

Nursing Care for AVF and AVG

Nursing care for arteriovenous fistula (AVF) and arteriovenous graft (AVG) is vital for successful hemodialysis. Preoperative care requires patient education about the procedure, consent acquisition, and confirmation of blood sample collection for investigative purposes. Vital signs should be monitored. Preoperative orders, such as prophylactic antibiotics and adjustments to antihypertensive drugs, should be carried out.

Postoperative care involves close monitoring for complications. The wound site should be observed for bleeding, hematoma formation, changes in color, swelling, and signs of infection. The AVF/AVG site should be kept clean and dry. Specific care includes assessing the patency of the vascular access by palpating for a thrill and auscultating for bruits. Checking the strength of the radial pulse, color, and warmth of the limb with the AVF/AVG is essential to ensure adequate blood flow. Hypotension during or after hemodialysis can cause thrombosis, so increasing the dry weight for the first 2-4 weeks after AVF/AVG is important. Elevation of the limb after the procedure helps in minimizing edema. Adequate pain management should also be provided.

Patient education is necessary for maintaining the functionality and health of the AVF/AVG. Patients should regularly check for thrill or bruit. They should avoid constrictive clothing, heavy loads on the affected arm, and extreme temperatures. They must also avoid letting anyone perform procedures or administer drugs in the access arm. Gentle exercises on the access arm can aid in the maturation of the AVF and increase awareness of the fistula. Keeping the access clean at all times is essential. Any signs of infection should be promptly addressed.

Cannulation techniques require careful inspection, palpation, and auscultation of the AVF/AVG prior to cannulation. Proper skin preparation should minimize infection rates. Local anesthesia may be administered for pain-sensitive patients. Proper needle site rotation is required to prolong the lifespan of the fistula and prevent pseudo-aneurysm formation. Needle gauge selection depends on vessel size. Smaller needles are initially used, and larger ones are used for high blood flow. In the cannulation of an arteriovenous fistula (AVF) for hemodialysis, the arterial needle (which draws blood from the patient) is placed downstream from the anastomosis site, while the venous needle (which returns blood to the patient) is placed further away from the arterial needle, generally upstream. The venous needle should be positioned at least 5 cm away from the arterial needle and angled in the direction of venous flow toward the heart. This technique aims to prevent recirculation.

Table 6: Types of Cannulation

Types of cannulation	Description	Rationale	Disadvantage
1. Rope Ladder Technique	Equal distribution of punctures along the whole length of the fistula in a systematic manner.	A long segment of the vein is required.	Small dilation over the whole fistula.
2. Buttonhole Technique	Every cannulation must be inserted into the same needle tract in the same direction, depth, and angle.	When there is a short segment of the vein. Self-cannulation.	Increased rate of infection.
3. Area Puncture	Repeated puncture of one or two sites.		Increased risk of aneurysm with stenosis in adjacent regions.

Appropriate documentation of every cannulation procedure is vital for future reference and continuity of care.

Nursing Care for Catheter Access

The preoperative preparation and postoperative follow-up for immediate complications such as bleeding and signs of infection are similar to AVF/AVG procedures. However, additional steps must be taken for cuffed, tunneled, percutaneous, and vascular catheters placed in the internal jugular and subclavian veins. After insertion, a chest X-ray should be performed. The image must be checked to confirm the correct positioning before use.

Vascular catheters carry a more significant infection risk, so infection prevention should be emphasized. The catheter exit site must be meticulously cleaned according to standard care and dressed using a sterile procedure with transparent dressings. A non-touch technique should be used when handling the catheter and capped and uncapped before and after use. Regular examinations of the catheter site must be conducted to check for signs of infection. Chlorhexidine or povidone-iodine is used to clean the catheter exits.

Blockage is a common problem with catheters and causes reduced flow rates and ineffective dialysis. Adequate flushing of the catheter and using a heparin lock can often prevent this issue. Continuously checking the insertion date for patients with temporary catheters is important. This is to avoid using the access for longer periods than intended, as this can increase the rate of complications.

Proper education on catheter care is necessary for patients. Nurses should guide them on maintaining the cleanliness and dryness of the catheter exit site. Patients should avoid exposing the site to water during activities and use a waterproof dressing before bathing. They should also ensure that clamps are closed and caps are in place when the catheter is not in use. This is to prevent potential complications. Patients must understand that pulling the catheter can cause dislodgment and should refrain from doing so. Any pain, swelling, or bleeding should be promptly reported to the staff.

Chapter 10: Dialysis Procedure

Principles of Hemodialysis

In the hemodialysis process, anticoagulated blood is pumped through an extracorporeal circuit. It passes through a biocompatible semi-permeable membrane which is called the dialyzer or 'artificial kidney' and is then returned to the patient's circulation. Within the dialyzer is a flow of ultrapure dialysate in the opposite direction that interacts with the patient's blood. Small solutes can traverse the membrane through diffusion, which is driven by concentration gradients, but larger molecules like cells and high-molecular-weight proteins remain restricted from crossing. A transmembrane pressure is applied to enable the controlled removal of fluids through ultrafiltration, which also aids in the removal of more solutes through convection.

Steps Involved in Hemodialysis

Before hemodialysis can be started, a vascular access point must be established. This can be done through arteriovenous fistula creation, an arteriovenous graft, or a catheter. The recommended placement choices for an AV fistula usually start with the wrist, (specifically the radial-cephalic fistula at the wrist) and then move up the arm if needed.

An AV graft is a surgically created artificial connection between an artery and a vein that is used as an alternative to an AV fistula. It is used when the patient's blood vessels are unsuitable for direct connection through the AV fistula.

The dialysis machine is set up and checked for proper functioning. The parts of the machine include a dialyzer, a filter, and a tubing system that carries the blood to and from the patient. The patient's vital signs, weight, and medical history are reviewed to determine the appropriate treatment procedures for the patient.

If an AV fistula or graft is in place, two needles are inserted into it (one to draw blood from the patient and the other to return the filtered blood to the patient's circulation). Catheters usually have separate ports for the same purpose.

Blood is pumped from the patient's body through one side of the dialyzer into the machine. Inside the dialyzer, the blood flows through numerous tiny hollow fibers, where waste products and excess fluids are filtered out, and the filtered blood is then returned to the patient's body via the returning tube and needles.

A special fluid that contains electrolytes is circulated on the other side of the hollow tube counter-currently to the patient's blood. This is known as the dialysate. This fluid helps remove waste products and excess fluid from the blood. As blood and dialysate flow in opposite directions through the dialyzer, waste products, toxins, and excess fluids are transported across the membrane into the dialysate. At the same time, essential substances like erythrocytes and proteins remain in the blood. During the dialysis session, the patient's vital signs, electrolyte levels, and overall clinical condition must be continuously monitored.

The dialysis machine can be adjusted to maintain the desired balance of fluids and electrolytes in the patient's body. After the dialysis session, the patient's vital signs are re-evaluated, and any complications or concerns should be addressed.

Hemodialysis is performed multiple times per week. Each session lasts several hours in accordance with the patient's specific needs. This process helps remove waste and excess fluids from the blood, similar to the kidneys' natural function, and helps patients with kidney failure manage their condition.

Understanding the Diffusion Process

Hemodialysis operates on the principle of solute diffusion through a semi-permeable membrane. The movement of metabolic waste products occurs along a concentration gradient from the bloodstream into the dialysate solution. Several factors influence the rate of diffusive transport, which include the magnitude of the concentration gradient, the membrane's surface area, and the membrane's mass transfer coefficient. The latter factor depends on the membrane's porosity and thickness, the solute molecule's size, and the fluid flow conditions on both sides. By the laws of diffusion, larger molecules exhibit slower transfer rates through the membrane. For instance, a small molecule like urea (60 Daltons) experiences significant clearance. Although larger molecules are generally cleared less efficiently in hemodialysis compared to smaller ones, creatinine (113 Daltons) is still effectively cleared through the process.

Ultrafiltration and Its Importance

The removal of water and sodium occurs via ultrafiltration rather than diffusion. Application of a negative pressure gradient on the dialysate side of the semi-permeable membrane achieves ultrafiltration.

Patients may accumulate excess fluid during hemodialysis between sessions, which can cause conditions like fluid overload and hypertension. Ultrafiltration helps to address this issue through the removal of the accumulated fluid from the patient's bloodstream into the dialysate. This process maintains the patient's fluid balance and prevents complications associated with fluid retention.

Isolated ultrafiltration represents a variant of ultrafiltration where no dialysate is employed, and the diffusion process is absent. Isolated ultrafiltration primarily removes water and does not significantly remove small molecular weight substances like urea. Unlike standard hemodialysis, where both solutes and water are removed, isolated ultrafiltration focuses on removing excess fluid, with minimal impact on the serum concentration of solutes like urea. The rate at which solutes are removed in isolated ultrafiltration is not equivalent to water and is limited due to the absence of a concentration gradient that is typically established by dialysate in standard hemodialysis.

Dialyzer Selection

Hemodialysis comprises three key components: the dialyzer, dialysate composition and delivery, and the blood delivery system. Dialyzers are the core components of the hemodialysis machine. This facilitates the exchange of solutes and fluids between the patient's blood and the dialysate solution. Various dialyzers are available, and the selection of an appropriate one depends on several factors. The dialyzer commonly used in the US uses hollow-fiber technology and allows simultaneous high-flow circulation of blood and dialysate. Modern dialyzers in the United States primarily use biocompatible synthetic membranes derived from materials like polysulfone, which is a shift from older cellulose membranes known for complement cascade activation. The global practice of reprocessing and reusing hemodialyzers and bloodlines varies. In the United States, disposable supplies have increased, making dialyzer reprocessing exceptionally rare. Various agents, like formaldehyde, peracetic acid-hydrogen peroxide, glutaraldehyde, and bleach, have been utilized for reprocessing.

An ideal dialyzer should have the following features: adequate ultrafiltration ability, negligible loss of proteins and amino acids, non-toxic compositions, reliability, minimal blood volume, minimal activation of cell or thrombotic pathway, and low cost.

Factors That Influence Dialyzer Selection

Several patient-specific factors and clinical considerations influence the choice of a dialyzer. These include the patient's medical history, comorbidities, vascular access, prescribed treatment duration, and anticipated treatment goals.

Additionally, the healthcare team considers factors such as the biocompatibility of the dialyzer material, the clearance of specific solutes, and the potential for complement activation. The goal is to select a dialyzer that provides optimal treatment and also minimizes the risk of adverse reactions and complications.

Types of Dialyzers

Coil dialyzers

Coil dialyzers are constructed with a cellulose acetate membrane tightly wound around a plastic or metal coil enclosed within a rigid plastic housing. These dialyzers were the earliest commercially available and mass-produced versions of the 1950s. Coil dialyzers had significant limitations such as a large priming volume, unpredictable ultrafiltration, and a high incidence of blood leaks.

Parallel plate dialyzers

Parallel plate dialyzers are constructed with layers that resemble a sandwich. Membrane sheets are positioned between support plates with ridges, grooves, or crosshatches. This setup facilitates membrane support and dialysate flow. Blood flows through these membrane sheets with a small, contained blood volume and modest heparin requirements. However, a drawback of parallel plate dialyzers is their compliance. Their blood-holding volume increases with higher transmembrane pressure (TMP).

Hollow-fiber dialyzers

Hollow-fiber dialyzers represent the predominant type used in contemporary practice. These dialyzers comprise a bundle that contains approximately 10,000 to 15,000 hollow fibers encased within a plastic sheath. Each fiber possesses a diameter that ranges from 200 to 300 micrometers. Blood is directed through these hollow fibers, while the dialysate circulates outside the fibers and follows a counter-current pattern. Hollow-fiber dialyzers maintain a shallow blood volume relative to their surface area due to their specific flow geometry. They offer minimal resistance to blood flow due to their numerous blood passages. Hollow-fiber dialyzers, like other dialyzer types, can exhibit some degree of compliance. This means they may slightly change shape or volume under varying transmembrane pressure (TMP). This characteristic allows for precise ultrafiltration control, and they are well-suited for reuse.

Dialyzer membranes

Semi-permeable membranes facilitate the filtration of waste products and excess fluids from a patient's blood. A dialysis membrane must possess specific qualities like high solute and water permeability, wet-state mechanical strength, biocompatibility, and cost-effectiveness. When exposed to blood, hemodialysis membranes experience dimensional changes and require exceptional mechanical strength. The ideal hemodialysis membranes are characterized by large pores, strength, flexibility, thinness, and low weight. Examples of the available semi-permeable membranes include:

- Cellulose-Based Membranes: These early hemodialysis membranes are derived from natural cellulose. They are biocompatible and effectively remove waste while maintaining electrolyte balance. However, they may activate complement and clotting systems in some patients.

- Synthetic Polymeric Membranes: These types are made from synthetic materials such as polysulfone, polyethersulfone, and polyacrylonitrile, not polyethylene. They offer improved biocompatibility, which reduces adverse reactions. They also precisely control pore size and permeability for toxin and fluid removal.

- High-Flux Membranes: With larger pores, high-flux membranes efficiently remove middle-sized molecules like beta-2 microglobulin and offer great benefits to chronic kidney disease patients.

- Low-Flux Membranes: Smaller-pored low-flux membranes are gentler and used in acute kidney injury or gentle dialysis treatments. They are, however, less efficient for larger molecules.

- Modified Membranes: Specialized membranes like heparin-coated ones reduce clotting risk.

Dialysate

The dialysate is a specialized solution formulated to support waste product removal and electrolyte balance during treatment. The potassium concentration in the dialysate can range from 0 to 4 mmol/L, dependent on the patient's pre-dialysis serum potassium levels. The use of extremely low potassium dialysate, such as 0 or 1 mmol/L, is less common. This is due to concerns about the increased risk of sudden death, which has been found to be linked with potassium shifts that cause arrhythmias.

The dialysate contains 1.25 mmol/L (2.5 mEq/L) of calcium, although adjustments may be necessary in certain situations. For instance, patients with hypocalcemia related to secondary hyperparathyroidism or "hungry bone syndrome" following parathyroidectomy might require higher dialysate calcium concentrations.

The standard dialysate sodium concentration falls within the range of 136–140 mmol/L. In cases where patients frequently experience hypotension during dialysis, "sodium modeling" may be employed to counterbalance urea-related osmolar gradients. Sodium modeling in hemodialysis typically involves initially using a higher dialysate sodium concentration, which may then be gradually reduced as the session progresses. However, the initial concentration is not as high as 145–155 mmol/L. However, it is essential to note that higher dialysate sodium concentrations and sodium modeling can cause a positive sodium balance and increased thirst. Therefore, these approaches to management of intradialytic hypotension may not be suitable for patients with hypertension or significant interdialytic weight gains.

Patients are exposed to approximately 120 liters of water during each dialysis session. The water used for dialysate undergoes a series of treatments like filtration, softening, deionization, and reverse osmosis in order to eliminate microbiological contaminants and dissolved ions.

The composition of the dialysate solution is carefully adjusted based on the patient's specific needs and laboratory values. The goal is to achieve and maintain a balanced electrolyte profile during dialysis and prevent rapid shifts that could cause complications like arrhythmias or muscle cramps. It is essential to monitor and adjust the dialysate composition as needed in order to ensure patient safety and treatment efficacy.

Monitoring the Dialysis Process

To ensure the safety and effectiveness of this treatment, it is essential to continuously monitor the hemodialysis process. This includes the following:

- Vascular Access Monitoring: An important aspect of hemodialysis monitoring is having adequate vascular access. This may involve assessment of the functionality of arteriovenous fistulas, grafts, or central venous catheters.

- Hemodynamic Monitoring: Continuous hemodynamic monitoring is performed during dialysis to assess the patient's blood pressure, heart rate, and any signs of hemodynamic instability. Hypotension (low blood pressure) is a common complication during hemodialysis, and prompt intervention helps to prevent adverse events.

- Ultrafiltration and Fluid Balance: Monitoring fluid removal prevents over-hydration or dehydration. The ultrafiltration rate is closely monitored to align with the patient's prescribed fluid removal target. Frequent adjustments may be required based on the patient's response and fluid status.

- Electrolyte and Biochemical Monitoring: Frequent blood sampling monitors electrolyte levels of sodium, potassium, calcium, and phosphorus. These parameters should be monitored to ensure that the patient's electrolyte balance is maintained within a safe range. Additionally, biochemical markers like urea and creatinine are tracked to assess the effectiveness of waste product removal.

- Dialysate Monitoring: The dialysate composition is continually monitored to maintain the desired electrolyte balance and achieve adequate solute clearance. The dialysate's temperature, conductivity, and pH are checked to ensure quality.

- Anticoagulation Monitoring: Anticoagulation is often required to prevent blood clotting within the dialysis circuit. Parameters like activated clotting time (ACT) or heparin dosage should be monitored in order to prevent clot formation and excessive bleeding.

- Dialyzer Reuse and Maintenance: In facilities where dialyzers are reused, stringent protocols for cleaning and disinfection are followed. It is crucial to monitor the dialyzer's integrity and functionality in order to prevent potential complications.

- Patient Comfort and Safety: Regular communication with the patient is vital during the dialysis process. Comfort level, and assessment for any discomfort should be monitored in order to contribute to a positive patient experience, and concerns should be addressed promptly.

- Documentation and Record-Keeping: Detailed and accurate documentation of the dialysis process is essential for patient care and regulatory compliance. Healthcare providers record vital signs, medications administered, and any complications observed during dialysis.

Post-Dialysis Assessment

After a dialysis session, a post-dialysis assessment is conducted to ensure the patient's stability. This includes evaluation of their vital signs, fluid status, and overall well-being.

Monitoring the hemodialysis process is a multifaceted and important aspect of providing safe and effective care to patients with kidney disease. It involves a comprehensive approach that encompasses pre-dialysis assessment, vascular access monitoring, hemodynamic stability checks, fluid balance management, and electrolyte monitoring. The diligent efforts of healthcare providers and the use of advanced monitoring technologies are fundamental to the achievement of the best outcomes for hemodialysis patients.

Complications of Hemodialysis

Like most medical procedures, certain complications of hemodialysis may arise. This complication can be acute or chronic. Complications include:

- **Dialysis disequilibrium syndrome:** This usually follows a rapid clearance of substances such as urea from the blood and can cause the accumulation and imbalance of fluid in the brain. Patients usually present with headache, confusion, nausea, restlessness, coma, and even death.

- **Hypotension:** Hypotension is the most common acute complication associated with hemodialysis, particularly in individuals with diabetes mellitus. Several factors increase the risk of hypotension in these patients. These factors encompass excessive ultrafiltration without sufficient compensatory vascular volume replacement, impaired vasoactive or autonomic responses, osmolar shifts, overuse of antihypertensive medications, and reduced cardiac reserve. Patients with arteriovenous fistulas and grafts may occasionally develop high-output cardiac failure due to blood diversion through dialysis access. In rare instances, this may require the surgical closure of the fistula or graft. Management of hypotension during the dialysis procedure usually involves discontinuance of ultrafiltration, administration of 100–250 mL of isotonic saline intravenously, or, in some cases, consideration of salt-poor albumin. Administration of salt-poor albumin for managing hypotension during hemodialysis can be available in outpatient settings, depending on the facility's protocols and resources. While not routinely used due to cost and other considerations, it is an option that can be considered in certain clinical situations in both inpatient and outpatient dialysis settings.

- **Infection:** Infections represent a significant cause of heightened morbidity and mortality in hemodialysis patients. The primary source of infection in hemodialysis is related to access sites. Additional areas of infection risk include pneumonia, skin, and soft tissues. These infections usually result from lapses in infection control measures, such as inadequate hand hygiene, cross-contamination of medical instruments, mishandling of intravenous medications, improper disinfection of dialysis equipment, and non-compliance with infection prevention and control protocols.

- **Air embolism**: During cannulation and in the process of hemodialysis, air leaks may occur via the dialysis tubing. Patients usually present with chest pain, breathlessness, cough, and orthopnea.

- **Hemolysis:** When red blood cells circulate through the hemodialysis circuit, they can undergo shear stress and form fragments. In addition, the dialysate contaminants and blood osmotic changes can worsen the breakdown oof red blood cells.

- **Allergic reaction:** This can be classified into Type A and Type B allergic reactions. Type A allergic reactions occur within 5-25 minutes during a hemodialysis session. They can range from pruritus, bronchospasm, and urticaria to anaphylactic shock. Type B allergic reactions usually occur later and are delayed. Type B allergic reactions, also known as delayed hypersensitivity reactions, are more likely to present with symptoms like a rash, fever, or joint pain, and they typically occur hours to days after exposure to the allergen. Chest or back pain should prompt an investigation into other more likely causes.

Other complications that may arise include vascular access hemorrhage and thermal burns. Hemodialysis is expensive and can significantly affect the financial security of families undergoing this routine. It can also affect patients' quality of life and waste a valuable amount of time each week just to undergo this procedure.

Prevention of Hemodialysis Complications

The critical care nurse must observe carefully before, during, and after the hemodialysis procedure to prevent complications.

Hemodialysis is a treatment modality for the management of end-stage renal disease (ESRD) symptoms. It enhances patients' overall quality of life. However, extended periods of hemodialysis can cause various complications as listed above. In order to mitigate the "legacy effects" of delayed treatment, renal transplantation should be considered for patients in early ESRD stages or before initiation of renal replacement therapy (RRT). Early detection and management of hemodialysis-related complications help to minimize mortality risk.

Many hemodialysis-related complications are highly preventable when addressed promptly, especially for infections, cardiovascular disease (CVD), vascular access problems, and dialysis disequilibrium syndrome. In order to ensure the well-being of patients who undergo hemodialysis, it is imperative to implement regular viral screening, vaccination, meticulous care of hemodialysis access, rigorous infection control protocols, effective anemia management, control of hypertension and diabetes, and diligent follow-up. Additionally, preservation of residual kidney function is essential.

Intradialytic hypotension can often be prevented through careful assessment of dry weight and ultrafiltration modeling. Instead, it typically involves a gradual and consistent removal of fluid throughout the session to prevent rapid changes in blood volume. It is essential to avoid excessively rapid fluid removal (over 13 mL/kg per hour) as it has been associated with adverse outcomes, which include cardiovascular deaths. Other strategies to prevent intradialytic hypotension include sequential ultrafiltration before dialysis, cooling the dialysate during treatment, and refraining from the consumption of heavy meals during dialysis.

Chapter 11: Hemodialysis Equipment and Components

Overview of Hemodialysis

Hemodialysis is a process that filters metabolic waste and excess water out of the blood. This is achieved by passing the blood through a machine with a special filter that acts as an artificial kidney. The filter has a semipermeable membrane that allows waste products and fluid to move from the blood, which has a higher concentration of these substances, into a cleansing fluid called dialysate. The unwanted substances cross the membrane until the concentrations on both sides are balanced, which effectively removes them from the bloodstream.

Hemodialysis is a form of renal replacement therapy for end-stage renal disease, and it can be used in acute kidney injury or disease as well. This treatment creates an access point in the patient's bloodstream, either through a surgically made passage that is known as a fistula or via an arteriovenous graft. Once the access is established, the patient's blood is circulated through a dialysis machine. Inside the machine, a semipermeable membrane allows waste products and any excess fluids to pass from the blood into a cleansing solution (known as dialysate), which is on the other side of the membrane. The transfer of solutes during hemodialysis occurs along a concentration gradient, not against it. In hemodialysis, waste products and excess electrolytes move from an area of higher concentration in the blood to a lower concentration in the dialysate. Then the dialyzed blood is pumped back into the patient's circulation.

Different factors, such as the concentration gradient magnitude, membrane surface area, and membrane mass transfer coefficient, affect the rate of diffusive transport. This depends on the membrane's porosity and thickness, the solute molecules' size, and the flow conditions on either side of the membrane. Small solutes move across the membrane faster (e.g., urea), while a larger molecule (like creatinine) is cleared less efficiently. Waste can be moved from circulation into the dialysate through ultrafiltration. Ultrafiltration utilizes convective removal to remove excess water from plasma, while solvent entrainment eliminates heavier substances. Dialysis lasts three to six hours and is done at least three times per week.

Overview of Dialysis Machine Components

The machine has multiple detectors, controllers, monitors, and safety devices that ensure safe operation. This allows the operator to control the blood and the dialysate circuits and monitor variables such as ultrafiltration, rate, adequacy, dialysate composition, and circuit pressures. There are three essential components to hemodialysis: the blood delivery system, the dialysate, and the dialyzer.

Blood Delivery System

The blood supply system has extracorporeal vessels and the ability to filter blood. The dialysis machine comprises a blood pump, a dialysis solution delivery system, and various safety monitoring devices. The blood pump moves blood from the access site through the filter to the patient. Blood flow usually ranges from 250–450 mL/min depending on the type and integrity of the vascular access. The negative hydrostatic pressure on the dialysate side can be adjusted to achieve the desired liquid removal or ultrafiltration effect. Hemodialysis membranes have different ultrafiltration coefficients and hydrostatic changes, so the amount of fluid removed may vary. The dialysate delivery system dilutes the dialysate concentrate with water and monitors the dialysate's temperature, conductivity, and flow rate. The blood supply system has the following components:

- Pressure monitors (arterial, pre-pump, and venous post dialyzer).
- Blood tubing.
- Blood pump.
- Heparin pump.
- Air leak detector.
- Clamps.

Arterial Pressure Monitor (Pre-pump)

This monitors the pressure between the blood line and the blood pump. The arterial pressure monitor measures the pressure in the arterial line that leads to the dialysis machine and is usually negative, and reflects the suction effect of the blood pump. It does not become positive after the blood pump. Alarms from this screen indicate patient disconnection, blood flow separation, or blockage. The negative pressure index in this segment makes it easy for air to enter the blood. When pressure is out of range, the blood line clamp activates and the alarm is triggered.

Venous Pressure Monitor (Post-dialyzer)

Venous pressure increases due to the venous return resistance between the intravenous drip chamber and the venous needle. The venous blood pressure monitor reads a positive pressure. Therefore, any pressure outside the allowable range will cause the blood line to clamp and stop the blood pump. This triggers appropriate alarms as well as closure of the venous return.

Blood Tubing

Biocompatible and non-toxic materials are used to make blood tubes. Silicone treatment is commonly used for blood tubing in hemodialysis to minimize clotting and is not rare in single-use systems.

Blood Pump

Peristaltic pumps are used in hemodialysis machines to pump blood through tubing at a flow rate of 200–600 mL/min. The pumps have two rollers powered by a low-voltage motor (to reduce the electrical risk). The blood pump is equipped with a spring to prevent insufficient or excessive blood tube blockage. The pump is adaptable to tubing of various sizes and can be operated manually in the event of a power failure. It is calibrated to measure blood flow based on the internal diameter of the tube.

Heparin Pump

The heparin pump, which can be a syringe or roller pump, infuses heparin into the blood circuit and not directly into the blood vessel.

Air Leak Detector

Air leak detectors in a hemodialysis machine are placed in the venous line.

Blood Tubing Clamps

Blood tubing clamps in hemodialysis machines are designed to withstand pressures associated with the blood circuit, but a specific pressure tolerance like 800 mmHg is not a standard specification for these clamps. In the event of a break in the circuit or electrical power loss, the blood tubing clamps deploy automatically. They can be opened manually in case of power loss.

The Dialysate System

Hemodialysis machines typically use a recirculating filtration system for dialysate. The provision of safe dialysate includes careful regulation of temperature, concentration, flow rate, pressure, and sterilization. Key components of the dialysate system include:

- Heating
- Deaeration
- Proportioning
- Monitoring
- UF (ultrafiltration)
- Disinfection

Heating the Dialysate

Most dialysis machines heat the dialysate to body temperature, which is approximately 98.6°F (37°C), not 92–102°F. This heating function improves dialysate mixing. The heating elements are stainless steel (not copper). This function is monitored downstream by the dialysate temperature controller in the dialysis circuit.

Dialysate Deaeration

The removal of water-soluble gases from the dialysis solution is important because their presence can cause gas embolism in the patient, not just flow problems. It may also impair the functionality of other monitoring and ultrafiltration devices. Air removal in dialysate deaeration is achieved through the application of negative pressure. Negative pressure is achieved by tightening the valve above the pump to circulate the water using an air trap and vent. Degassing in dialysate preparation is usually not achieved by heating water to 185°F. This temperature is excessively high for standard deaeration processes in dialysis machines.

Dialysate Proportioning

The term "dialysate dosage" is not typically used. The correct term is "dialysate proportioning," which involves mixing treated water with concentrate to achieve the desired composition, temperature, and conductivity. This is achieved using metering pumps and concentrates.

The Dialyzer

This is also known as an artificial kidney. It is a chamber capable of perfusing blood and dialysate at high flow rates. Blood and dialysate flow in opposite directions in the dialyzer to optimize the efficiency of diffusion and filtration.

Classifications of Dialyzers

Dialyzers are classified into low-flux and high-flux categories, where the distinction is based on their permeability and ultrafiltration rates.

Low-flux membrane dialyzers (type I) — These dialyzers have an ultrafiltration rate of less than 15 mL/mmHg/h and a beta 2-microglobulin clearance rate of less than 15 mL/min. Low-flux membrane dialyzers excel at filtering out small molecules from the blood with ease. However, when it comes to midsized molecules, which can be toxic and are typically more challenging to eliminate through the diffusion process, these dialyzers achieve moderate removal effectiveness.

High-flux membrane dialyzers (types II and III) — These dialyzers have an ultrafiltration rate of ≥15 mL/mmHg/h and a beta 2-microglobulin clearance rate of ≥15 mL/min. They feature high hydraulic permeability and higher permeability for middle-sized solutes. They can remove large molecular weight beta 2-microglobulin as well as other macromolecular substances.

Protein-leaking membranes improve anemia, reduce total plasma homocysteine concentrations, and reduce glycosylated plasma and oxidized protein concentrations.

High-performance hemodialysis machines utilize advanced filtration technology and incorporate a range of synthetic membranes. These include the polysulfone membrane series for their durability and biocompatibility, polyacrylonitrile membranes that are known for their high permeability, polymethylmethacrylate membranes that are selected for their ability to remove particular toxins, and cellulose acetate membrane dialyzers, which are traditional membranes used in various treatments.

Types of Dialyzers

Hollow fiber dialyzers — Hollow fiber filters are the most commonly used. These dialyzers consist of bundles of capillary tubes through which blood flows while the dialysate flows outside the bundle.

Parallel plate dialyzers — Do not necessarily have a larger surface area than hollow fiber dialyzers. They are often used for pediatric patients but not specifically because they have a larger surface area or due to limited space. Dialysate and blood circulate through flat plates with small channels.

Tube dialyzers — Blood and dialysate circulate around semipermeable tubes instead of fibers like those previously discussed. They are not as common as hollow fiber and parallel plate dialyzers.

Biocompatibility of Dialyzers

Biocompatibility describes the compatibility of the materials and design of a dialysis machine with the patient's blood. Dialysis machines commonly use polysulfone or polyether sulfone membranes. These materials are less likely to trigger an immune response or cause adverse reactions in patients. Some dialyzers are designed to minimize complement system and neutrophil activity, which can lead to inflammation and other side effects. Synthetic fiber membrane filters in dialyzers are made from materials like polyacrylonitrile, polymethyl methacrylate, polysulfone, polycarbonate, polyethylene, and polyamide.

Cellulose acetate is a specific type of cellulose membrane used in dialyzers. It's not that cellulose's biocompatibility is strengthened by mixing it with acetate; rather, cellulose acetate is a distinct material used for its properties.

Reuse of Dialyzers

Dialyzers reuse has declined in some developed countries. The main reasons are concerns about patient safety and infection control. The practice varies based on regional policies, economic factors, and healthcare infrastructure. Reuse of dialyzers requires strict cleaning, sterilization, and quality control procedures to ensure the safety of patients. With such measures in place, a dialyzer can be used for twelve to twenty-four sessions before being replaced.

Dialysate Composition and Preparation

Dialysate typically contains glucose, but not always at physiological levels. The glucose concentration in dialysate can vary and is sometimes omitted depending on the patient's needs. It circulates in the water tank of the hemodialysis machine to control the diffusive transport of small molecules across the membrane and achieve the desired blood concentration. Dialysate commonly has six electrolytes: potassium, sodium, calcium, magnesium, chloride, and bicarbonate. Glucose (dextrose) is a common component in dialysate.

The table below shows components of the dialysate and their concentrations in millimoles per liter (mmol/L). The values reflect a range. They may vary based on an individual patient's requirements.

Table 7: Components of dialysate

Component	Concentration (mmol/L)
Sodium	135–145
Potassium	2–4
Calcium	1.25–1.75
Magnesium	0.25–0.375
Chloride	98–124
Bicarbonate	25–35
Glucose	0–11
pH	7.4

Dialysate potassium concentrations range from 0–4 mmol/L (depending on the initial serum potassium concentration). The use of dialysate potassium at 0 or 1 mmol/L has become rare because patients dialyzed with very low dialysate potassium concentrations are at increased risk of sudden death, possibly due to arrhythmias from changes in potassium levels.

The calcium concentration in the dialysate can vary. Although 1.25 mmol/L is a common concentration, it's not the standard for all dialysate formulations. An adjustment may be necessary in some instances, such as in patients with hypocalcemia associated with secondary hyperparathyroidism after parathyroidectomy (who may require higher calcium concentrations in the dialysate).

The sodium concentration in the dialysate can vary widely, and ranges from 135 to 145 mmol/L, as mentioned earlier in the text. Sodium concentrations in patients with frequent hypotension during dialysis are slightly lowered to isotonic concentrations. This is done near the end of dialysis treatment and is called sodium modeling or profiling. Higher sodium concentrations and modeling may result in a positive sodium balance, which is undesirable in hypertensive patients or those who gain weight between dialysis sessions.

Preparation of Dialysate

The dialysate buffer can be prepared on-site or off-site in a pharmaceutical lab. The water used must be treated to prevent contamination and other unwanted dissolved ions. The water treatment involves filtration, softening, deionization, and reverse osmosis to remove microbiologic contaminants and dissolved ions. Once the water is treated, bicarbonate is added in proportions denoted as acid: base: water. After the base buffer is made, components such as potassium, sodium, calcium, magnesium, chloride, and glucose are added per Table 7. The dialysate is tested for bacteria endotoxin, and the pH is measured and maintained at 7.4. It is then stored in sterile containers or bags before use and continuously monitored for quality control.

Chapter 12: Complications and Adverse Events

Hypotension

This is the most common acute complication of hemodialysis, with an incidence of 15–30%. It is characterized by decreased systolic blood pressure of about greater than 20-30 mmHg from predialysis pressure, or systolic blood pressure of less than 100 mmHg. It is more common in older patients and women.

Etiopathogenesis

Many factors contribute to the development of hypotension. The removal of large volumes of plasma results in reduction of the intravascular volume, which reduces the hydrostatic pressure that causes hypotension. This mechanism is similar to that of anemia and dehydration. Thermal energy transfer from the dialysis machine causes vasodilation and resultant hypotension. Autonomic dysfunctions have also been found in patients on hemodialysis. The use of antihypertensive medications, especially within 4 hours of commencing dialysis, may precipitate the development of hypotension. Endstage renal disease patients with underlying cardiac diseases such as myocardial infarction and arrhythmias have a higher tendency to develop hypotension. Dialyzer reaction, anaphylaxis, and septicemia by way of causing vasodilation through generation of vasoactive substances and inflammatory mediators, can also cause hypotension. Other causes of hypotension include air embolism and electrolyte derangements such as hyponatremia and hypocalcemia.

Clinical features

The clinical findings in hypotension will depend on the underlying cause. The common symptoms found are low blood pressure, tachycardia/bradycardia, cold clammy extremities, pallor, seizures, altered consciousness, dizziness, blurring of vision, headache, muscle cramps, yawning, and generalized body weakness.

Management

The management of hypotension depends on the underlying cause. General measures include decreasing dialysate temperature for suspected thermal energy transfer. Midodrine can be used to reduce the risk of hypotension during dialysis. Its administration should be based on clinical judgment and patient-specific factors. It's not a universal recommendation for all patients who undergo hemodialysis. Putting the patient in the Trendelenburg position increases the venous return to the heart, which increases the cardiac output and results in improved tissue perfusion. Infusing 200–500 mL of 0.9% saline or 100 mL of 20% albumin increases the oncotic pressure with increased blood pressure. Decreasing the ultra-filtration rate will reduce the rate plasma removal.

Other measures such as increasing the dialysate sodium and calcium concentration have been found to reduce the risk. The use of short-acting antihypertensives, especially vasodilators within 4 hours of dialysis, should be minimized.

Muscle cramps

Muscle cramps occur in about 5–20% of hemodialysis sessions. It causes significant patient discomfort and occasionally results in the termination of hemodialysis.

Etiopathogenesis

Multiple causes have been identified to cause muscle cramps. Factors or conditions that will result in intravascular volume depletion or cause rapid removal of sodium or hyponatremia can result in muscle cramps.

Clinical features

Clinical features of muscle cramps can occur at any time during hemodialysis but it is more common especially at the middle of end of dialysis. These signs and symptoms mostly involve cramping of the extremities.

Management

Muscle cramps respond well to a single bolus of normal or hypertonic saline. Pharmacologic agents such as quinine sulfate, diazepam, vitamin E, and carnitine have been used successfully. Decreasing the ultrafiltration rate and increasing estimated dry weight has been beneficial.

Headache

Etiopathogenesis

Headaches can be caused by several factors, ranging from hypertension, hypotension, excessive fluid removal, rapid fluid and electrolyte shift, anxiety, and tension.

Clinical features

Patients usually complain of pain in the head or facial area. Other features will depend on precipitants.

Management

Analgesics are the hallmark of management in addition to treating precipitants such as antihypertensives for hypertension and normal saline infusion for hypotension.

Dialysis disequilibrium syndrome

This is a set of neurologic and systemic symptoms of varying severity that occur primarily due to cerebral edema in dialyzed patients. It occurs most frequently within the first few dialysis sessions in new patients who have high BUN levels.

Etiopathogenesis

Rapid change in solute concentration and pH in the central nervous system causes fluid to shift into the brain due to the removal of wastes from the bloodstream. This results in cerebral edema, which has been proposed by two theories: the reverse osmotic shift induced by urea removal and a fall in intracellular pH. Rapid changes in serum electrolytes, especially in new patients, have also been implicated.

Clinical features

Usual findings include headache, nausea, disorientation, restlessness, blurring of vision, and asterixis. More severe patients develop confusion, seizures, coma, and even death. Some strategies to reduce disequilibrium syndrome are the use of smaller surface-area dialyzers, reduction of rates of blood and dialysate flow, high dialysate sodium, and intravenous administration of diazepam.

Management

Dialysis disequilibrium syndrome symptoms are self-limiting and usually resolve within hours. The management of mild nonspecific disequilibrium symptoms, such as nausea, vomiting, restlessness, and headache, is symptomatic. However, in the acutely uremic patient with such symptoms who is undergoing dialysis, the blood flow rate should be slowed, and consideration should be given to stopping the dialysis session. Dialysis is stopped in the patient with seizures, coma, and obtundation. Severe dialysis disequilibrium syndrome with seizures can be reversed more rapidly by raising the plasma osmolality with either 5 mL of 23% saline or 12.5 g of hypertonic mannitol.

Chest pain

Etiopathogenesis

Chest pain is also a common complication with several causes. Chest pain that occurs during dialysis could be associated with hypotension or hypovolemia. Factors also include dialysis disequilibrium syndrome, angina, myocardial infarction, hemolysis, rapid blood flow rate, and pulmonary thrombo-embolism. The other predisposing factors were discussed earlier.

Chest pain in angina is caused by myocardial ischemia and is usually relieved by nitroglycerin. It should always be considered in patients with an increased risk of coronary artery disease. Appropriate history and physical examination should be carried out. Electrocardiogram and cardiac enzyme evaluation should be performed.

If the dialysis is to be continued, the administration of oxygen, nitrates, or morphine, and the reduction of the ultrafiltration speed should be considered on an individual basis.

Instead, these medications are used carefully considering their potential effects on blood pressure and dialysis efficacy. The main consideration is the balance between managing angina and maintaining adequate blood pressure during dialysis.

Clinical features

This includes pressure or pain that can be localized or may radiate to neck, jaw, shoulders, and arms. It may wax and wane, which usually lasts by 1–2 minutes. Some complain of choking, squeezing, and crushing chest sensation. Others complain of nausea, pallor, and cool clammy skin.

Chest pain caused by myocardial ischemia can often be relieved by nitroglycerin, especially in cases of angina. Nitroglycerin helps by dilating blood vessels and reducing the heart's workload. However, in the case of myocardial infarction, where there is actual necrosis of heart tissue, relief with nitroglycerin may be less effective or not effective at all.

Chest pain of myocardial infarction occurs with chest pain that is localized or radiates to the neck, jaw, and shoulders; arms that may come and go; apprehension; choking sensation; squeezing; crushing sensation; nausea pallor; cool, clammy skin; and hypotension.

The hemodynamic status of the patient and the clinical findings will determine if the hemodialysis should be stopped or continued.

Management

The management options include treatment of angina pain with nitroglycerin. Myocardial infarction pain with analgesics and hypotension was discussed earlier.

It can be prevented by accurate fluid removal and weight assessment.

Arrhythmia

Arrhythmias are abnormal rhythms of the heart characterized by irregular and uncoordinated electrical activity. It can be either harmless or life-threatening. Common types include atrial/ventricular fibrillation, supraventricular tachycardia, and premature contractions.

Etiopathogenesis

Both patient and hemodialysis factors contribute to the risk of arrhythmias. Cardiac disease associated with conduction disturbances such as atrial and ventricular ectopy are known to cause arrhythmias. Changes in extracellular fluid ion composition, rapid extracellular fluid volume fluxes, rapid lowering of potassium and other electrolyte disturbances such as hypomagnesemia and hypocalcemia may precipitate arrhythmias. Some cardiac drugs such as digitalis commonly used in hemodialysis patients are arrhythmogenic.

Clinical features

Arrhythmias can present as palpitations, tachycardia/bradycardia, chest pain, shortness of breath, dizziness, lightheadedness, and even syncopal attack.

Management

The dialysis procedure should be stopped unless there is a clear metabolic precipitant that can be corrected by dialysis (e.g., hyperkalemia-induced heart block). Intravenous access via the fistula or central line should be maintained. Life-threatening rhythms should be managed according to advanced cardiovascular life support (ACLS) guidelines. Aggressive ultrafiltration can indeed exacerbate arrhythmias and should be avoided. Discontinuation of arrhythmogenic drugs or conversion to other alternative and aggressive medical and surgical therapy of underlying cardiac diseases have been beneficial in the management of arrhythmias.

Cardiac arrest

It is a sudden cessation of cardiac activity and a rare but life-threatening medical emergency that requires immediate intervention and can occur at any point in time. Several factors have been implicated in patients on hemodialysis.

Etiopathogenesis

Cardiac arrest is associated with multiple causes. However, the most common causes in relation to hemodialysis are fluid and electrolyte imbalances, arrhythmias, dialysis disequilibrium syndrome, and underlying cardiac disorders.

Clinical features

The features are those of absent pulses, absent cardio-respiratory activity, cessation of breathing, loss of consciousness, and unresponsiveness.

Management

Cardiopulmonary resuscitation and defibrillation is the immediate intervention while underlying causes are addressed. Monitoring of patients' vital signs, electrolyte levels, and overall clinical condition during dialysis is especially important. Adjustment of the dialysis prescription can minimize the risk of rapid fluid and electrolyte shifts.

Air embolism

This is the presence of air into the extracorporeal system that spreads into the systemic circulation. It is a potentially fatal complication of hemodialysis.

Etiopathogenesis

Potential sources of venous air embolism are the arterial site, improperly connected and loose bloodlines, disconnected central venous catheters, empty IV bags, air leaks in blood lines, and unarmed air detector connections.

Intravascular air is more likely to cause reduction of cerebral perfusion, resulting in focal neurologic symptoms. It is particularly important to monitor and ensure optimal functioning of devices on the dialysis machine.

Clinical features

Patients with air embolism can present a pink foamy air pocket in the extracorporeal system venous line, cough, shortness of breath, chest pain or pressure, tachycardia, distended neck veins, and cyanosis. There may also be weakness or paralysis of one side of the body, confusion, convulsions, and even coma.

Management

The management of suspected air embolism involves clamping of the venous line and stopping the blood pump, positioning of the patient on the left side in a supine position with the chest and head tilted downward, provision of cardio-respiratory support, and the administration of 100% oxygen by either a mask or endotracheal tube.

Air embolism can be prevented. Keep the level of drip chambers up, replace empty saline bags immediately, tighten connections when priming, tape needles securely, and follow correct priming procedures.

Dialysis-related amyloidosis

Etiopathogenesis

Dialysis-related amyloidosis is specifically characterized by the deposition of beta-2 microglobulin-derived amyloid (AB2M) in bones and joints. It occurs more commonly in patients who have been on long-term hemodialysis and affects osteoarticular structures.

Clinical features

There are a variety of clinical presentations depending on the type, site, and amount of amyloid deposition. Most common symptoms include joint stiffness, pain and swelling, numbness or tingling in the hand and finger, weakness in the hand muscles, painful skin nodules or plaques, fatigue weight loss, and malaise.

Amyloid protein deposition and retention are attributed to the type of dialysis membrane, prolonged uremic state, decreased dieresis, increased advanced glycation end products, elevated levels of cytokines, and the type of dialysate.

Management

Require close monitoring of these patients. Provide adequate and optimal hemodialysis and analgesics for pain and inflammation. Institute surgical interventions where necessary.

Dialyzer reactions

These are allergic reactions that occur in a patient on hemodialysis. Two forms have been described. These are the first-use syndrome and the dialyzer membrane hypersensitivity.

Etiopathogenesis

First-use syndrome is not necessarily an IgE-mediated anaphylactic reaction but rather a type of hypersensitivity reaction. It usually occurs within 20 minutes of starting hemodialysis. Effects are reproducible during subsequent sessions.

Hypersensitivity to the membrane is a reaction to cellulose and or polymethylmethacrylate, which are components of the dialyzer membrane.

Clinical features

These features may include urticaria, pruritis, hives, angioedema, dyspnea, hypotension, wheezing, and chest tightness.

Management

Stop the dialysis once there is an anaphylactic response, and treat it with epinephrine and steroids.

Pyrogenic reaction

Etiopathogenesis

This is a febrile reaction due to the presence of dead bacteria and/or endotoxins within the systemic circulation. Low molecular weight endotoxin fragments may be able to cross any membrane irrespective of membrane pore-size distribution and contaminate the containers, distilled water machine, dialyzer, and the bloodlines.

Infection or septicemia from contamination of bicarbonate containers/system, water system, machine, dialyzer, or bloodlines is a common identifiable cause. However, cold dialysate can make the patient shake and shiver without fever.

Clinical features

Patients with pyrogen reactions usually do not develop a cold sensation upon initiation of dialysis. The symptoms of a pyrogenic reaction, such as chills and fever, usually occur during or after dialysis. There may be sudden shaking chills, followed by temperature elevation within 1--2 hours after chills. Tachycardia, hypotension, headache, and muscle aches are also present.

Management

When pyrogen reaction is noticed, the dialysis should be immediately suspended and the patient should be assessed. Intravenous fluid, antipyretics, and antibiotics are used in the management. Pyrogenic reactions can be prevented by proper disinfection/sterilization and the use of aseptic techniques.

Itching

Etiopathogenesis

This is caused by dry skin; secondary hyperparathyroidism; abnormal levels of calcium, magnesium, and phosphorus in tissues; allergies; and elevated blood urea nitrogen.

Management

Management involves adequate dialysis to regulate electrolyte levels. Provide lotions or medications for dry skin.

Infections

Infection in patients with hemodialysis is a significant cause of morbidity and mortality. The most common source of infection is access-site–related infections. Infection transmission can occur at any time but typically occurs during the start or at the end of the hemodialysis session. Patients on hemodialysis are at a greater risk of bloodborne infections.

Etiopathogenesis

Many factors contribute to infection whereas others are the main sources of infection in hemodialysis. Factors such as improper hand hygiene, cross-contamination of instruments, mishandling of intravenous medications, inadequate disinfection of dialysis equipment, poor or nonadherence to infection prevention and control standard practices, and suppressed immunity have been found to be common among dialyzed patients with infections.

Bacterial pathogens include *Staphylococcus aureus***,** coagulase-negative staphylococci (CONS)**,** *Pseudomonas aeruginosa***,** *Escherichia coli***,** *Klebsiella,* and *Enterobacter*. viruses such as the hepatitis B virus (HBV), hepatitis C virus (HCV), and HIV are common. Although Candida and Aspergillus species can cause fungal infections in hemodialysis patients, these are not usually the predominant types of infections. Bacterial infections are more common, particularly with Staphylococcus aureus.

Clinical features

Infections have a wide range of manifestations and can vary depending on the type. Some common features include fever, fatigue, malaise, inflammation, nausea, vomiting, and headache.

Management

Identify organisms and treat them appropriately by administering the appropriate antimicrobials and providing supportive management.

Infections can be prevented by observing infection control practices and good hand hygiene, proper dialysis equipment, environmental hygiene, adequate vascular access care, judicious use of antibiotics as indicated, and prophylaxis for immune-compromised patients.

Electrolyte derangement

These are electrolyte disturbances commonly seen in patients on hemodialysis. The most common of these electrolyte disturbances are hypo/hyperkalemia, hypo/hypercalcemia, hypo/hypernatremia, and hypomagnesemia.

Etiopathogenesis

Electrolyte imbalances in hemodialysis are caused by multiple factors such as excessive removal of electrolytes from the blood during dialysis, dietary restrictions, medications such as phosphate binders, and longer or frequent sessions that can cause significant electrolyte derangements.

Clinical features

The clinical features of electrolyte derangement depend on the electrolyte that is deranged. Hyponatremia may present with nausea or vomiting, muscle weakness, and cramps. Headache, confusion, altered mental status, seizures, or coma may also occur. Hypernatremia clinical features include increased thirst, dry mucous membranes, restlessness, confusion, seizures, and coma.

The clinical features of hypokalemia include muscle weakness and cramps, constipation, arrhythmias, and muscle paralysis. Clinical features of hyperkalemia are muscle weakness, tingling or numbness, muscle twitching or cramping, nausea or vomiting, and diarrhea.

Hypocalcemia can manifest with muscle cramps, spasms and weakness, numbness and tingling sensations, tetany, or seizures. Hypercalcemia can manifest with excessive thirst and frequent urination, constipation, confusion, depression, or altered mental status, and muscle weakness.

Management

Electrolyte levels assay and ECG monitoring should be done. Pharmacological management of derangements and adjustment of dialysate electrolyte concentrations are beneficial, along with dietary restrictions.

Hypertension

Etiopathogenesis

Some factors such as fluid overload increase the hydrostatic pressure, resulting in elevated blood pressure. Noncompliance with blood pressure medications, anxiety, and renin overproduction are known to affect blood pressure significantly.

Clinical features

Hypertension may begin gradually or suddenly. This resuts in headache, blurring vision, nausea or vomiting, dizziness, and seizure.

Management

Treatment includes administration of antihypertensive medications and an assessment of target weight and fluid removal goal.

Clotting

Etiopathogenesis

This is the formation of blood clots in the dialyzer and blood lines. Clotting may be attributed to inadequate anticoagulation, low blood flow rate, poor priming techniques, and loose connections.

Clinical features

This includes increased venous pressure readings, visualization of dark blood in lines or drip chambers visualization of fibrin in drip chambers, and visible clots or clumps of dark blood in the drip chamber or dialyzer.

Management

The management is mostly anticoagulation and resolving the underlying cause.

Hemolysis

Hemolysis involves the breakdown or destruction of red blood cells, and there is a decrease in the oxygen-carrying capacity of the blood. It is potentially life-threatening because severe hyperkalemia can lead to cardiac arrest.

Etiopathogenesis

The etiology of hemolysis in hemodialysis patients is usually related to multiple causes. These include mechanical factors such as poorly functioning or incorrectly calibrated blood pump, excessive negative pressure in the extracorporeal circuit, deformity in lines (kinks, folds, etc.), and over-occlusion of the blood pump. Chemical factors are delivery of improperly prepared dialysate, contamination of dialysate with chemical agents such as formaldehyde, bleach, chlorine, copper, nitrates, and nitrites, and hypotonicity due to an insufficient concentrate-to-water ratio. Although overheated dialysate can contribute to hemolysis, the threshold temperature is generally considered to be higher than 42 degrees Celsius (107.6 degrees Fahrenheit).

Clinical features

Clinical features include complaints of chest pain, shortness of breath, and/or back pain. Finding port wine appearance of blood in the venous line is highly suggestive of hemolysis. A falling hematocrit and a pink color of the plasma in centrifuged specimens are also indicators.

Management

The management is to stop the dialysis immediately and clamp the blood lines, and then do a rapid potassium and other electrolyte assays. Also, prepare to treat hyperkalemia and anemia. Hospitalization and observation are paramount because life-threatening hyperkalemia may develop after dialysis has been terminated.

Nausea and Vomiting

Etiopathogenesis/Management

The most common causes are hypotension, uremia, and disequilibrium syndrome. Treatment of the underlying cause or precipitant and pharmacological management with antiemetics for intractable cases will address this complication.

Chapter 13: Nutritional Considerations

Patients who undergo hemodialysis are at a high risk of malnutrition, which could range from mild to severe. This nutritional state presents with deficiencies in calories, protein, and other important macro- and micro-nutrients. Consequently, hemodialysis patients are prone to protein-energy wasting. The latter is defined as an inappropriate supply to meet the body's need for calories and protein. For this reason, a special nutritional management plan is indispensable for patients with chronic kidney disease (CKD) on hemodialysis.

Recent guidelines recommend that patients on maintenance hemodialysis should have a protein intake of at least 1.1 grams per kilogram of ideal body weight (IBW) per day. To achieve this goal, hemodialysis patients are obligated to follow a strict diet that supplies sufficient fluids and nutrients. In general, the diet should consist of adequate calories, high protein and vitamins, and low potassium and sodium.

Research demonstrates the vital role of dialysis nurses in improving patient outcomes through education about their illness and the importance of nutrition. For instance, nurses are advised against the use of harsh or judgmental tones when a patient presents with complications due to dietary indiscretion. With that said, a tailored nutritional plan requires the expertise of a certified dietician. This is further emphasized by studies that showcase the low number of hemodialysis patients who have an adequate intake of calories and protein. The majority of patients consume less than 35 kcal/kg/day, whereas more than 20% have a protein intake of less than 1 g/kg/day.

Healthcare providers should educate patients on selecting protein sources that are appropriate for their individual dietary needs. They should consider the level of phosphorus, potassium, and sodium content. More specifically, an emphasis on the phosphorus/protein ratio should be placed. Ideally, patients should choose meats with low phosphorus and fat but high protein. A daily portion of meat and eggs is essential for a healthy diet. However, it may not be sufficient for patients on hemodialysis. This is where nutritional supplementation becomes helpful. These supplements help achieve target protein and energy intake.

The first type is oral nutritional supplements, which supply the body with enough amino acids to maintain the patient's muscle mass and provide tissues with necessary building blocks. A meta-analysis demonstrates that oral supplementation increases serum albumin levels by an average of 0.23 g/dL without adverse effects on electrolytes. The administration of oral supplements during hemodialysis is practical and well-tolerated.

There is also some evidence that oral supplementation can improve the outcome of hypoalbuminic patients on hemodialysis.

The second supplementation option is intradialytic parenteral nutrition (IDPN), which is preferred for patients who cannot tolerate oral supplements. The benefits of IDPN mostly revolve around the anabolic effects seen in patients. Clinicians should favor oral intake when possible.

The adherence of hemodialysis patients to adequate nutritional guidelines requires a close follow-up with a certified dietician who has clinical experience with nephrology patients. Additionally, physicians and nurses should attempt to communicate to patients the importance of strictly following these guidelines without the use of punitive tones when complications related to poor adherence arise.

Chapter 14: Psychosocial Aspects of Hemodialysis

Chronic kidney disease can take a significant toll on the patient's mental and emotional well-being. Approximately 25% of hemodialysis patients exhibit symptoms of depression, whereas anxiety affects slightly fewer patients. However, some reports place the incidence of anxiety and depression in hemodialysis patients on the upper end (up to 45%). Depression is a common mental disorder in hemodialysis patients that significantly impacts treatment adherence, admission rates, and quality of life.

One interesting aspect that plays a role in the response of patients to hemodialysis is religion. Religious and cultural beliefs seem to alter the way patients perceive the suffering and challenges associated with hemodialysis, which may contribute to a positive outcome.

The transition to hemodialysis can be very challenging psychologically. Patients will express negative feelings about future uncertainty, financial strain, physical dysfunction, and lifestyle changes. The transition can be severe enough to trigger denial, regret, depression, anxiety, and isolation. Initially, patients may be non-compliant with dietary guidelines and fluid restrictions. Denial can lead to withdrawal, which increases the risk of adverse effects. Beyond the initial phase, patients may undergo identity alterations due to changes in body image and dependence. Therefore, healthcare providers must realize the importance of the first year of hemodialysis in the process of adaptation and acceptance.

Hemodialysis may also have a negative impact on social interactions, personal relationships, and professional careers. In fact, patients will commonly switch jobs and settle for lower-paying positions. Depression and social isolation may persist until the patient fully accepts the new treatment. The transition from other therapeutic modalities to hemodialysis may also be psychologically daunting. For instance, patients face difficulties transitioning from peritoneal dialysis to hemodialysis.

All these aspects should highlight the importance of psychosocial care during hemodialysis, especially in the initial phase. Regular assessments of psychological status with a patient-centered approach, along with social and emotional support, are recommended. Nurses should establish trust with patients to help them develop healthy coping mechanisms.

Various screening measures can be used to assess the mental health of hemodialysis patients. These include the Beck Depression Inventory, Patient Health Questionnaire, and Hospital Anxiety and Depression Scale. These measures are recommended throughout the treatment period. The complexity of depression diagnosis in dialysis patients is acknowledged, especially in consideration of the overlap of symptoms with uremia and the influence of comorbid conditions.

The management of depression in hemodialysis patients is therefore critical to prevent poor treatment adherence and morbidity. Management includes pharmacological and nonpharmacological interventions. Pharmacological treatment primarily involves antidepressant drugs, such as selective serotonin reuptake inhibitors (SSRIs). Fluoxetine and sertraline are among the most commonly prescribed SSRIs. They cause fewer side effects compared to tricyclic antidepressants. Other classes of antidepressants such as selective norepinephrine reuptake inhibitors (SNRIs) and monoamine oxidase inhibitors are less preferred due to their heavy side effect profile.

Chapter 15: Infection Control

Infection control is essential in hemodialysis units to ensure the safety of patients and reduce the financial toll caused by infections. Due to the close contact of nurses with patients, it is vital to follow antiseptic measures in order to reduce the incidence of infections.

Infection control precautions

During the hemodialysis process, there is a high chance of exposure to microbes that lead to epidermal and dermal infections.

Glove usage

Healthcare providers must wear disposable gloves during care for hemodialysis patients. This also applies to those who handle the equipment used for hemodialysis. Therefore, a steady supply of non-sterile gloves at each dialysis station is indispensable. The gloves are disposed after each procedure which lowers the risk of contamination. Sterile gloves are used for procedures that require a sterile environment, such as catheter insertion and certain aspects of arteriovenous fistula or graft care. Without appropriate measures, bacteria from the surface of the skin can cause severe infections. The most common pathogen that causes surface infections in hemodialysis patients is Staphylococcus aureus. The level of sterility required for these procedures mandates the use of sterile gloves.

Hand hygiene

Aside from glove usage in hemodialytic procedures, healthcare providers should also pay attention to hand hygiene. Hands should be thoroughly washed after removal of the gloves and between patient contacts. To facilitate this process, each hemodialysis unit should have several sinks with warm water and soap to allow nurses and other healthcare professionals to wash their hands frequently. Alternatively, a waterless antiseptic can be suitable if the hands are not soiled.

Hand hygiene focuses on two components to lower the risk of microbial transmission. These are hand washing and hand antisepsis. The former is the act of cleansing one's hands with soap and water, which becomes very important when the hands are soiled with contaminants. Hand antisepsis means the use of sanitizers to reduce the bacterial load on the hands of the healthcare provider. Many medical workers have a misbelief that gloves replace proper hand hygiene. This could contribute to the infections seen in hemodialysis patients. Clearly, proper hand hygiene is a requisite in the case of aseptic procedures.

There is also some evidence that highlights the importance of hand hygiene beyond healthcare providers. Patients and their family members should follow proper hand hygiene protocols when entering the dialysis room. This comprehensive approach to hand hygiene is essential to minimize infection transmission.

Item handling

Many items are introduced to the patient's dialysis station, including needles, catheters, charting tools, and personal belongings. These items could potentially be hosts for all sorts of microbes. They could also be contaminated with blood and body fluids. If an item is intended for single use, it should be disposed of directly after the hemodialysis session. Other items should be cleaned and disinfected to avoid exposure of infectious pathogens to other patients.

Medication handling

Intravenous medication ampoules labeled for single use should not be punctured more than once. The usage of these ampoules compromises their sterility. Furthermore, it's important to prepare medications in a separate area designated for medication preparation. Medications should be delivered individually to each patient. However, the use of common carts to distribute medications within the treatment area is discouraged. If a hemodialysis unit uses trays for the individual delivery of medications, they should be cleaned to prevent cross-contamination.

Blood contamination prevention

The reuse of these filters is not a standard practice and is discouraged to prevent cross-contamination and infection. It is vital to replace these items to lower the risk of blood contamination of the dialysis machine pressure monitors. Proper disinfection of the dialysis stations between patients is also important. Close attention should be paid to the control panels on the dialysis machines and other surfaces that are frequently touched by patients. The thorough cleansing of fluids and the disinfection of surfaces and containers (e.g., attached buckets) is also recommended.

To handle dialyzers intended for reprocessing, it's essential to cap dialyzer ports as well as clamp tubing. Used dialyzers should be placed in leakproof containers to facilitate safe transport from the station to the reprocessing area.

In case of blood spills, it is necessary to clean with an appropriate disinfectant. For cleaning blood spills in a healthcare setting like a dialysis unit, a 1:10 dilution of household bleach (5,000-6,000 mg/L free chlorine) is recommended. A 1:100 dilution (300-600 mg/L free chlorine) is weaker and may not be sufficient for effectively disinfecting blood spills, which require a stronger solution to ensure the elimination of bloodborne pathogens. The staff member who cleans the area should wear gloves. Also, the used cloth should be placed in a leakproof container. After removal of visible blood, apply disinfectant again with a new cloth.

Personal protective equipment

Healthcare staff should wear personal protective equipment (PPE), such as gowns, face shields, eye protection, or masks when they perform procedures with a risk of blood spatter. These protective measures are not only for the safety of staff but also to prevent contamination of patients. Staff should be vigilant and change protective clothing if it becomes soiled. It should be prohibited to eat, drink, or smoke in the dialysis treatment area to maintain a sterile environment. However, patients can be served meals or have food brought from home with standard cleaning practices applied to glasses, dishes, and utensils.

Cleaning and disinfection

Written protocols

Dialysis units should have written protocols to clean and disinfect surfaces and equipment. Mechanical cleaning should be carried out before any disinfection process.

When available, follow the manufacturer's instructions for sterilization or disinfection of equipment. This includes the adherence to appropriate dilution and contact time recommendations for chemical sterilants and disinfectants.

Environmental surfaces

After the hemodialysis session, environmental surfaces at the dialysis station should be cleaned. This includes the dialysis chair, countertops, and external surfaces of the dialysis machine (e.g., containers). The use of standard soap or detergent germicide is recommended. For reusable medical equipment, mechanical cleaning followed by disinfection is vital. In the case of visible contamination with blood, a tuberculocidal disinfectant is appropriate.

Water treatment

Cleanliness and disinfection should also extend to the water treatment, distribution system, and the internal circuits of the dialysis machine. These methods not only control bacterial contamination but also eliminate bloodborne viruses. The cleaning procedures should be conducted according to evidence-based methods. For single-pass machines, the disinfection process should be done at the beginning or end of the day. Batch-recirculating machines should be drained and disinfected after each use. The same procedures apply in the event of a blood leak irrespective of the type of dialysis machine. Routine bacteriological assays of water and dialysis fluids should be conducted. The frequency and specifics of these assays should be based on the standards set by regulatory authorities and professional guidelines, such as the Association for the Advancement of Medical Instrumentation and the Centers for Disease Control and Prevention.

Venous pressure transducer protectors

Venous pressure protectors should be used to cover pressure monitors. If the external protector gets wet, it should be replaced immediately. A thorough inspection includes an examination for possible blood contamination of the internal pressure tubing set and pressure sensing port. If contamination is found, the machine must be taken out of service and disinfected with bleach. Frequent bloodline pressure alarms or adjustments of blood drip chamber levels may be indicators of this problem. Individual incidents of equipment contamination should be reported immediately to the FDA due to their potential public health significance.

Waste management

Workers in the dialysis facility play an important role in maintaining a clean environment. Their most important role is to remove infectious waste and make sure that the environment optimizes patient care. All disposable items should be placed in designated bags to prevent leakage. Waste products from the dialysis facility should be considered infectious if they are contaminated with blood. These solid medical wastes should be removed through incineration or in a sanitary landfill in compliance with local and state regulations.

Isolation strategies

Infection control within dialysis units should also focus on effective isolation strategies to prevent the spread of infections from patients with suspected or confirmed infections.

These strategies aim to minimize exposure and transmission of infections among patients and staff within the dialysis unit.

Standard precautions to deal with all suspected or confirmed infections have been put in place. These precautions include the use of personal protective equipment (PPE), such as masks, face shields, gowns, and gloves, as soon as a clinical suspicion is present. In specific cases, additional precautions are necessary based on the mode of transmission (e.g., droplets, airborne).

Patients with infections who require contact preventive measures should be isolated in individual rooms. In the case of airborne infections, dialysis should ideally be performed in a negative-pressure room to prevent the spread of airborne particles. Note that inter- and intra-hospital transfers of patients who require isolation should be limited to only the most essential cases.

Infection control measures during the dialysis procedure

One of the key recommendations to prevent infections during dialysis is to minimize the use of temporary catheters and keep them in place for the shortest necessary period. They also should be removed as soon as a permanent vascular access (e.g., arteriovenous fistula, graft) is available. This approach is essential to reduce the risk of infections associated with catheter use.

It is also important to regularly examine the catheter exit site and catheter hub for signs of infection when patients use catheters for dialysis. Inflammatory signs include warmth, redness, and swelling at the site of the catheter. This approach ensures that infections are identified and addressed early.

During the manipulation of catheters, healthcare providers are advised to wear masks and sterile gloves. This is vital to prevent the transmission of infections. For patients with arteriovenous access, vascular access site care is key. It may also be useful to wash the vascular access site with antibacterial soap and water before cannulation.

Chapter 16: Medical Management of the Dialysis Patient

Adequate or Optimal Dialysis Prescription and Delivery

Adequate or optimal dialysis is the minimum acceptable dose administered to a dialysis patient to prevent significant mortality and morbidity. It is the key to increasing the survival rate of the patient. For a patient to be categorized as optimally dialyzed, he must meet the following criteria:

Blood pressure before dialysis (predialysis blood pressure) should be less than 140/90 mm Hg. This criterion is the same regardless of whether the patient takes hypertensive medication.

Usually, important plasma concentrations to monitor include potassium, bicarbonate, and inorganic phosphate levels. This value is without the absorption of ion exchange resin. Furthermore, the value of bicarbonate should always be more than 24 mmol/l, and the inorganic phosphate level must be less than 1.6 mmol/l, which should be measured when the patient is not under oral binding agents. The hemoglobin level should be within 11.5-13 g/100ml.

Dialysis and Systemic Anticoagulation

Oral and systemic anticoagulants are one of the first-line drugs used during dialysis. Uremia can cause hemorrhagic complications like bleeding from the nose (epistaxis), purpura, and bleeding from the venipuncture site. Anticoagulants can prevent these anomalies. Its use to manage bleeding from venipuncture sites is controversial. Heparin can be used to prevent the bleeding the systemic anticoagulants. Furthermore, it inhibits clotting in the extracorporeal circuit.

Anticoagulation Therapy during Hemodialysis

During dialysis, blood flows through the extracorporeal circuit. This process activates the intrinsic pathway of coagulation, which, in turn, activates thrombin and fibrin. Due to the activation of this pathway, platelets adhere to the artificial surface of the dialyzer. The adhesion causes ATP to be released, which releases thromboxane A2 and other products. This initiates a coagulation cascade. The result of all this activation is the formation of a thrombus.

Heparin

Several anticoagulants, such as heparin and fondaparinux, have been implicated in minimizing thrombin formation during dialysis. Heparin and fondaparinux do have intrinsic anticoagulant properties. Heparin exerts its anticoagulant effect by binding to antithrombin, which then inhibits thrombin and other clotting factors. Heparin is one of the most commonly used anticoagulants in dialysis patients and is a nonuniform mixture of mucopolysaccharides. The molecular weight of heparin ranges from about 3,000 to 30,000 Da. It contains polymers of D-glucosamine-L-iduronic acid and D-glucosamine-D-glucoronic acid.

Actions of Heparin

Anticoagulant

Heparin exerts its anticoagulation property indirectly, as it is responsible for activating antithrombin. A heparin-antithrombin complex forms when heparin binds to antithrombin. This complex binds to clotting factors involved in various coagulation activation pathways. Some common clotting factors heparin inhibits are Xa, IXa, XIIa, and XIIIa. This makes heparin an effective anticoagulant agent both in vitro and in vivo.

Heparin does not activate factor VIIa. It is a factor involved in the extrinsic pathway of coagulation. Heparin administered at low doses can affect the conversion of prothrombin to thrombin. It can be concluded that the anticoagulant effect of heparin inhibits coagulation factors like Xa and the conversion of fibrinogen to fibrin. Therefore, fibrin, an end product of extrinsic and intrinsic coagulation pathways, does not get formed, which inhibits the coagulation pathway.

Antiplatelet

Heparin administered in higher doses can inhibit platelet aggregation, which increases bleeding time.

Lipemia clearing

Heparin is an effective lipemia-clearing agent. Heparin administered at a lower dose than used for anticoagulation can achieve this effect. When heparin is injected, it clears post-prandial lipemia. This action causes lipoprotein lipase to be released from the vessel wall, which in turn is responsible for the hydrolysis of triglycerides and very low-density lipoproteins.

Adverse Effects

1. The most common side effect of heparin is bleeding. This effect only occurs when administering heparin as an overdose rather than the usual requirement for dialysis. However, even with proper monitoring and ethical practice, one to three percent of patients can have serious bleeding. The first sign to appear is hematuria, so patients should carefully be assessed if bleeding is suspected.

2. The risk of osteoporosis is generally associated with higher doses and long-term therapy, which is less common in routine hemodialysis. This can cause pathological fractures and other manifestations. However, this effect only occurs when heparin is used in higher doses than normal.

3. Due to aggregation of platelets, mild thrombocytopenia can occur in patients who take heparin. Serious thromboembolic events can occur in these patients but are rare. In some instances, platelet levels can go down severely due to the formation of a complex of platelets and heparin, which should be managed by immediate suspension of heparin. Caution should be taken when using low molecular weight heparin in these patients and avoided as much as possible.

4. Hair loss, including alopecia, can occur during heparin use. Because alopecia caused by heparin is reversible and transient, treatment can continue despite these effects.

5. Under rare circumstances, hypersensitivity reactions to heparin can occur. The patient manifests with fever and urticaria and warrants urgent attention.

Contraindications

- Malignancy - These tumors usually have large and fragile feeding vessels. Heparin can cause significant bleeding in the necrosed part of the tumor and is very difficult to control.
- Tuberculosis - heparin may cause an increased incidence of hemoptysis.
- Subacute bacterial endocarditis - Heparin may increase the risk of embolism.
- Suspected and diagnosed gastrointestinal ulcers - Heparin always increases the risk of bleeding in such cases.
- History of severe hypotension - Heparin increases the risk of cerebral hemorrhage.
- Aspirin or any antiplatelet drug - Heparin increases the risk of hemorrhage, so these medications should be used with caution if needed.

- Thrombocytopenia - Heparin should be avoided as much as possible.
- Lumbar puncture - Heparin can cause subsequent bleeding, which is difficult to control.
- Ocular and neurosurgery - Heparin can cause bleeding, which is difficult to control.

  When a patient is undergoing dialysis, a bolus of heparin should be given before the process starts, i.e., the administration should occur before the patient is connected to the extracorporeal circuit. Heparin can be given under continuous infusion after the patient is connected to the extracorporeal circuit. There is no standard protocol for the amount of heparin administered. The dose is usually calculated based on the patient's age, sex, weight, and other guiding parameters. The dose should be adjusted based on clinical judgment throughout the process to prevent unwanted clotting or bleeding. Maintaining the dose of heparin and bleeding prevention is a double-edged sword and can only be achieved by careful monitoring and constant evaluation.

Guidelines for Heparin Administration in Hemodialysis

Guidelines have been created to ease the dose calculation and achieve the best coagulation profile in a dialysis patient. Initially, the patient should be given around 2,000-5,000 International Units of heparin. This dose can be given by opening a venous line or other access lines.

After administering the initial dose, it is important to wait two to three minutes so that the initial bolus mixes with the circulation uniformly. This is followed by continuous heparin infusion at 500-1,000 International Units per hour. This maintenance dose can be given by opening an arterial line.

During each of these processes, PTT is measured and monitored carefully. Hemodialysis sessions usually last for a few hours (around 4 hours).

The PTT guides the amount of heparin infusion during dialysis. For example, if PTT measured from the arterial line is more than forty-five seconds, the heparin infusion rate is decreased by 100 International Units per hour. Similarly, if PTT measured from the venous line is less than sixty-five seconds, the heparin infusion rate is increased by 100 International Units per hour. Furthermore, it is advisable to increase the heparin infusion by 200 International Units per hour if the arterial PTT is less than forty seconds.

Cryoprecipitate and Desmopressin

Cryoprecipitate impacts the coagulation profile of dialysis patients by increasing the vWF. Cryoprecipitate is a plasma product with an increased concentration of molecules such as fibrinogen, fibronectin, and vWF. It treats acute bleeding in uremia patients. Its effect has been implicated and used in various surgical and invasive procedures to decrease the bleeding rate. The use of cryoprecipitate and desmopressin in patients undergoing dialysis has been associated with significantly decreased bleeding time.

Management of Hyperkalemia

Due to the disturbance of normal renal homeostasis, hyperkalemia is one of the most common problems associated with patients with end-stage renal disease and in those undergoing dialysis. Acute hyperkalemia is defined as a potassium value of more than 6.5 mmol/l. It is considered an emergency, and the patient should receive immediate dialysis to prevent dreadful complications like ventricular fibrillation. In patients with life-threatening hyperkalemia, administration of intravenous salbutamol can be effective. Patients undergoing dialysis are advised to have strict dietary control and completely avoid potassium-rich foods to prevent hyperkalemia. Bicarbonate can also be used to correct the potassium level but is not as reliable for control.

Management of Hyperphosphatemia

Phosphate binders are the first line of treatment to manage hyperphosphatemia in patients with end-stage renal disease. Aluminum-containing phosphate binders were historically used to manage hyperphosphatemia in patients with end-stage renal disease. Their use has significantly declined due to concerns about aluminum toxicity, including encephalopathy and bone disease. However, they can cause aluminum toxicity and result in harmful side effects like myopathy and encephalopathy

In patients with end-stage renal disease, hyperphosphatemia can also develop secondary hyperparathyroidism and calcium deposition in sites other than bones (extraosseous sites) and should be managed accordingly.

With the advancement of medical science and recent drug delivery, calcium-containing compounds are now the most commonly used drugs for treating hyperphosphatemia. They should always be ingested with food to maximize the phosphate taken with each meal.

Control of Blood Pressure

Control of Hypertension

A dialysis patient with end-stage renal disease can develop hypertension. It is a common factor that can increase the incidence of mortality and morbidity due to the development of cardiovascular and cerebrovascular complications. Thus, hypertension needs to be strictly controlled. Antihypertensive medication in these patients is essential to manage their dialysis appropriately. Furthermore, patients should also be advised to maintain a strict diet to manage their blood pressure. The criteria for choosing and prescribing antihypertensive drugs should be rational and are described as follows:

- **Angiotensin-converting enzyme inhibitors (ACE inhibitors)**
  ACE inhibitors are one of the most commonly used drugs to control hypertension in a patient with end-stage renal disease. They are usually preferred if the patient also has left ventricular heart failure or endocrine manifestations like diabetes. It should be noted that anaphylactic reactions can occur in hemodialysis patients due to reactions with the AN69 membrane. This rare anaphylactoid reaction is unpredictable, and the group of antihypertensive drugs should be changed immediately if such reactions occur.

- **Angiotensin II receptor antagonists**
  In patients with hypertension who are undergoing dialysis for end-stage renal disease, monotherapy with angiotensin II receptor antagonists is a safe and effective alternative to angiotensin-converting enzyme inhibitors.

- **Calcium channel blockers**
  Calcium channel blockers do not affect leak or receptor-operated channels. They only block voltage-sensitive channels. These channels are normally present in the smooth muscle cells. This group of agents has maximum efficacy in patients with coronary heart disease. However, caution is advised when using them due to their potential additive effects on heart rate and the heart's contractility.

- **Beta blockers**
  In patients with coronary heart disease who are undergoing dialysis for end-stage renal disease, beta blockers are one of the antihypertensives that are safe to use. Beta blockers can be used concurrently with calcium channel blockers in certain clinical scenarios, including in patients with coronary heart disease who undergo

dialysis for end-stage renal disease. Alpha-adrenergic receptor blockers and other antihypertensive agents like nitroprusside can also control hypertension.

The dosing and frequency of the antihypertensive drug depend on several factors, which include a patient's status and weight. A stepwise protocol has been developed for the systematic use of antihypertensive medications in these patients and includes the following steps:

Step 1: The patient is treated with monotherapy, such as AT1-angiotensin II receptor antagonists, angiotensin-converting enzyme inhibitors, or beta blockers.

Step 2: A loop diuretic is added if urinary output in this patient is high, i.e., more than 600 ml. Furosemide is the most commonly used drug among the loop diuretics.

Step 3: If the blood pressure is not controlled or maintained within the targeted limit by the agents mentioned above, then a two or three-drug combination can be added. A calcium channel blocker can be added in this step.

Step 4: A bilateral nephrectomy is only indicated if all the mentioned drugs and therapy fail to control the hypertension.

Control of Hypotension

Dialysis causes a hypovolemic state in patients, and thus, cardiac output is limited. This can cause hypotension in these patients and should be managed accordingly. The most commonly implicated drugs in the management of hypotension are as follows:

(1) Midodrine

It is one of the most commonly used medications to control hypotension in dialysis patients and is an α-adrenergic agonist. It is available in the oral formulation and decreases intradialytic hypotension.

(2) Fludrocortisone

This medication has been shown to decrease intradialytic hypotension and can be an alternative drug to manage hypotensive patients on dialysis.

(3) Vasopressin

This drug can decrease intradialytic hypotension by constricting the splanchnic vessels. This action redistributes blood volume during fluid removal and can help manage hypotension in dialysis patients.

Management of Nausea and Vomiting

Nausea and vomiting occur in up to ten percent of patients with end-stage renal disease undergoing dialysis. Antiemetics like cyclizine and treatment of associated hypotension are usually sufficient to manage these patients.

Management of Headache

Headache occurs in up to seventy percent of patients with end-stage renal disease undergoing dialysis. Acetaminophen is prescribed for these patients.

Management of Anemia

Anemia is a frequent issue in patients with end-stage renal disease who are on dialysis. To treat this, recombinant human erythropoietin is commonly used, as it stimulates the production of red blood cells (erythropoiesis). The JAK-STAT pathway is involved in the signaling mechanism of many cytokines and growth factors, including erythropoietin, but erythropoietin itself does not bind directly to a JAK-STAT kinase-binding receptor.

Erythropoietin has significantly reduced the problem, but it has adverse effects. Some of the common adverse effects are listed below:

- Increased hypertensive episodes in dialysis patients.
- Increased clot formation in shunts.
- May act as a seizure-inducing agent.

Treatment with erythropoietin alone is sometimes not enough to correct anemia. This may be due to the following:

- Malignancy.
- Absolute or functional iron therapy.
- Inflammatory conditions.
- Aluminum overload.
- Sickle cell disease.
- Anti-epoetin antibodies.

Management of Infection

Many precautions and measures can prevent infections in dialysis patients. However, they do occur and will need medical management. Vancomycin and gentamicin are often used to manage infection in dialysis patients. Gentamicin is derived from the bacterium Micromonospora purpurea. It is one of the most commonly used drugs to treat infection in dialysis patients. However, its dose needs to be modified in cases of renal insufficiency. The modified dosing of gentamicin is summarized below:

- Give seventy percent of the daily recommended dose if creatinine clearance is 70 ml/min.
- Give fifty percent of the daily recommended dose if creatinine clearance is 50 ml/min.
- Give thirty percent of the daily recommended dose if clearance is 30 ml/min.
- In clinical practice, gentamicin dosing is individualized based on patient-specific factors, including renal function, and often involves therapeutic drug monitoring.
- Give forty percent of the daily recommended dose if creatinine clearance is <10 ml/min.

Antifungals like micafungin, echinocandin, and anidulafungin can be added if fungal infection is suspected.

Source: Adapted from Mermel LA et al. Clinical practice guidelines for the diagnosis and management of intravascular catheter-related infection: 2009 update by the Infectious Diseases Society of America

Management of Lipid Abnormality

Fibric acid analogs like gemfibrozil are commonly used drugs to manage lipid abnormalities in patients undergoing dialysis. It can lower the triglyceride level by activating peroxisome proliferator-activated receptor alpha. In the final run, this corrects the lipid abnormality in dialysis patients. However, in suspected or diagnosed cases of rhabdomyolysis, fibric acid should not be used in combination with statins.

Management with Calcitriol

Vitamin D is significantly reduced due to physiological disturbance in the kidney in dialysis patients with end-stage renal disease. These patients are treated with calcitriol, which is the active form of vitamin D.

Management of Secondary Hyperparathyroidism with Cinacalcet

Cinacalcet is a commonly used drug for the management of secondary hyperparathyroidism in cases of dialysis. It decreases the level of parathyroid hormone. This action is due to the activation of calcium-sensing receptors, which are normally in the parathyroid gland.

Prevention of Communicable Disease

Hepatitis B Virus Infection

Due to advancements in medical science, many preventative measures have been applied to protect dialysis patients with end-stage renal disease against the hepatitis B virus. Several vaccination protocols have been postulated to minimize the impact of hepatitis infections.

Hepatitis C Virus Infection

Hepatitis C is transmitted through blood transfusions or from the reuse of dialyzers. Preventive measures like disinfecting surfaces and disposal of instruments minimize the risk and help prevent hepatitis C virus infection.

Chapter 17: Peritoneal Dialysis

Approximately 3.8 million people worldwide require some form of renal replacement therapy for treating end-stage renal disease. When choosing the dialysis regimen, the patients and their doctor decide between peritoneal dialysis and hemodialysis. Peritoneal Dialysis is a form of dialysis treatment regimen used in patients with end-stage renal disease. The peritoneum's anatomy makes it a suitable membrane for solute diffusion and exchange. It is estimated that peritoneal dialysis is the method selected for around 11% of patients undergoing dialysis. This number varies in different countries. In some countries, peritoneal dialysis is the first method of choice due to its low cost and higher quality of life than hemodialysis patients. Peritoneal dialysis enables the patient to be more mobile and independent. Many patients prefer PD over hemodialysis because they can maintain their regular everyday activities and employment.

Peritoneal dialysis has certain clinical advantages and is often considered simpler to use than hemodialysis due to its home-based nature. Peritoneal dialysis may be associated with fewer hospital visits compared to in-center hemodialysis, but it is not necessarily associated with a lower overall infection risk. PD has its own specific infection risks, including the risk of peritonitis. However, it has some disadvantages, such as poor blood pressure control due to fluid overload, problems with the peritoneal dialysis machines, abdominal pain, and catheter care. The most critical complication of peritoneal dialysis is peritonitis. Because peritonitis has a high chance of mortality, the healthcare team should be educated on preventative and risk-reducing measures. You can find these measures in the International Society for Peritoneal Dialysis (ISPD) recommendations. Proper training of patients and their caregivers can minimize the rate of peritonitis and other potential complications.

Techniques and Procedures of Peritoneal Dialysis

When choosing peritoneal dialysis as the dialysis treatment regimen, there are certain issues that should be addressed. The clinician must ensure that the patient and his or her family are educated on the therapy's impact on their quality of life, the importance of maintaining proper hygiene, and the possible complications of PD. Other questions that need to be addressed are when to start dialysis, the timing of catheter placement, how to maintain volume control, the long-term viability of the therapy, and the dialysis dose to be targeted. After choosing peritoneal dialysis, the clinician selects between continuous ambulatory peritoneal dialysis (CAPD) and automated peritoneal dialysis (APD). Both regimens are home-based modalities that the patients themselves can perform. The main difference is that CAPD is performed manually, whereas APD employs a cycler, which is a mechanical device that assists the dialysate exchanges. Elderly patients with many comorbidities constitute the more significant proportion of patients on dialysis. These patients usually cannot perform the peritoneal dialysis independently or operate the cycler. Nurses must be well-trained and provide regular home visits to achieve the best outcomes for these patients.

Continuous Ambulatory Peritoneal Dialysis (CAPD) vs. Automated Peritoneal Dialysis (APD)

CAPD and APD are used in patients with end-stage kidney failure, but in some cases, one type of therapy is preferred. In the past, the main factor that influenced the peritoneal dialysis treatment regimen choice was the patient's peritoneal membrane characteristics. Dialysis patients are classified into high and low transporters based on the speed of solutes and fluid transport from the peritoneum. It is considered that high transporters have a more permeable peritoneal membrane. APD was used to be recommended only for high transporters due to its shorter dwell times, and it was avoided in low transporters. However, recently, it has been shown that APD can be used in all patients. This has contributed to the increase in the use of APD worldwide, especially in developed countries. However, APD is more expensive and has 20% higher costs than CAPD.

CAPD treatment faces several issues, such as the patient's lack of motivation, failures in technique, and increased risk of peritonitis. The risk of peritonitis can be reduced by using a double-bag format pre-attached to a Y-shaped transfer set of tubing. With this method, the patient is not required to connect the tubing to the fill bag. This method is called the "twin bag system."

CAPD treatment has been shown to alter the peritoneal membrane's structure and function. This may occur due to the recurrence of peritonitis and exposure to high concentrations of glucose contained in the solute. Some structural changes may include sub-mesothelial fibrosis, increased fibroblasts, and loss of mesothelial cells.

The risk of peritonitis in peritoneal dialysis can be influenced by several factors including patient training, technique, and adherence to aseptic procedures, rather than the mode of PD (APD vs. CAPD) itself. APD also reduces intra-abdominal pressures because it is done in the supine position compared to CAPD, which is done in the upright position. When looking at residual kidney function, the results are conflicting. Some studies reported that patients undergoing APD have a faster decline in residual kidney function, whereas others cannot prove this finding. There have also been reports in the literature that the removal of salt and water is lower in APD compared to CAPD, but the evidence is insufficient to make a conclusion.

Today, the main factors that drive the choice between these two modalities are quality of life and patient preference. Patients with active lifestyles, children, workers, and the elderly prefer APD over CAPD because they are free from intraabdominal fluids during the day. Patient preference increases compliance. Clinical conditions that should be considered when choosing between CAPD and APD are the presence of nonreducible hernias, loss of residual renal function (RFF) or ultrafiltration (UF), membrane characteristics, pre-existing slipped disc, and uterine and/or vesicle prolapse in women.

Insertion, Care, and Maintenance of Peritoneal Catheters

The Peritoneal Catheter

Before starting peritoneal dialysis, a catheter should be inserted in the abdominal cavity to allow for fluid transfer. Functional long-term access to the peritoneal cavity with a safe and durable peritoneal catheter is necessary for successful continuous ambulatory peritoneal dialysis. The peritoneal catheter can be placed with open surgical, laparoscopic, or percutaneous techniques. Most catheters are made from silicone rubber, a biocompatible and durable material. The catheter comes in various shapes such as straight, swan-neck, or pigtailed-curled. It can have a different length and number of Dacron cuffs used to anchor the catheter in the rectus abdominis muscle. The standard catheter has a double Dacron (polyester) cuff and comes in a straight or coiled tip with a straight or preformed arc-bend intercuff segment. Various types of peritoneal catheters are available, including one with a one-cuff, coiled-tip, and two-cuff extension catheters with preformed inner cuff bands. Many configurations of catheters have been made to address common mechanical issues such as tip migration, peri catheter leaks, and tissue attachment. These configurations have not demonstrated superiority over the standard design but are more costly and difficult to insert or remove.

Selecting the Most Suitable Catheter

Patients have different body sizes and shapes, comorbidities, and other needs that make it impossible for the catheter choice to be a one-size-fits-all approach. The peritoneal dialysis team should be educated on the various types of catheters to achieve peritoneal access tailored to the needs of the individual patient.

To achieve these goals, the team must consider the patient's body habitus, the presence of other acute or chronic conditions, and the dimension and shape of the catheter. Other factors that influence catheter choice include the patient's belt line, physical disability, hygiene habits, occupation, presence of intestinal stomas, gastrotomy tubes or suprapubic catheters, dermatologic conditions, and skin creases, folds, and scars.

Catheter Insertion

The catheter tip should be located in the true pelvis. The exit site location is ideally positioned in a zone with a low infection risk. The catheter insertion site and the length of the intraperitoneal tubing determine the pelvic position of the catheter tip. The site location should be visible and easily accessible by the patient. The patient should be able to easily insert the catheter through the abdominal wall without any tubing stress. To achieve proper placement of the tubing, it is recommended to use the pubic symphysis as the reference point for catheter insertion. Using the umbilicus as the reference point may lead to excessively deep placement, which may cause flow dysfunction and pain at the end of the effluent drain.

The exit site is the location on the abdomen from where the catheter comes out. The exit site of the catheter should be reachable from the location of the pelvic position. The exit site cannot be within the belt line, on the blind side or apex of an obese skin fold, or inside a crease. Extended catheters allow the exit site to be placed away from the lower abdomen to the upper abdomen, back regions, and the presternum. This can be used in patients with intestinal stomas, severe obesity, or multiple abdominal folds. Determining the insertion and exit site location can be made more accessible with the use of stencil-based preoperative mapping. Marking stencils can help professionals determine the most appropriate catheter type, as well as the ideal insertion and exit site location.

The selection of the most appropriate type of peritoneal dialysis catheter is not solely based on factors like the position of the patient's belt line or the presence of obesity, but rather on a comprehensive assessment of the patient's anatomy, medical condition, and lifestyle. A patient with a high-lying belt line benefits from a preformed, swan-necked, inner-cuff arc bend catheter with a downwardly directed exit site. A patient with severe obesity, multiple abdominal skin folds, intestinal stomas, or incontinence should receive an extended catheter with a presternal exit site.

A catheter inventory with all the items needed for the peritoneal access procedure and a protocol for preoperative mapping enables the peritoneal dialysis access team to provide the patient with the most appropriate catheter type and an optimal insertion and exit site location.

Catheter Implantation Techniques

Catheter implantation techniques include the percutaneous needle-guidewire technique, open surgical technique (mini-laparotomy), and laparoscopic techniques.

The percutaneous needle-guidewire is a convenient technique that can be done at the bedside under local or general anesthesia and prophylactic antibiotics. This technique is done with a prepackaged kit that includes the dialysis catheter. Ultrasonography and fluoroscopy can be used to guide the needle. This increases the safety of the technique. This technique is considered to be less invasive, but there is a risk of improper catheter placement and bowel perforation.

The open surgical technique is done under local, regional, or general anesthesia. This technique is known for its safety, simplicity, and good results. It is recommended for patients who receive a peritoneal catheter for the first time and those with no abdominal surgery history. Also, a previous abdominal surgery can be a consideration in the choice of technique for peritoneal dialysis catheter placement.

The laparoscopic technique is increasing in popularity. One of the reasons is that during this technique, the surgeon can perform partial omentectomy or adhesiolysis while placing the catheter. The laparoscopic approach is done under general anesthesia, with the patient placed in the supine position. With this technique, the surgeon can examine the abdominal cavity thoroughly, which allows for better catheter placement.

To successfully place the catheter, the team should be educated on the catheter placement techniques and possible complications such as dialysate leakage, exit-site infections, catheter malfunction, etc.

Catheter Care and Maintenance

Before finally placing the catheter, the access team should test the patency and flow function by doing a trial irrigation with a sufficient volume of solution. Postoperatively, the catheter should be flushed with 500- to 1 000 -mL volume dialysate or saline solution. This should be done weekly until dialysis is started. Flushing prevents obstruction by fibrin or blood clots. Flushing can also help the team detect possible catheter malfunctions. This enables them to intervene in a timely fashion. Peritoneal dialysis can be initiated two weeks after the catheter insertion procedure to avoid complications such as catheter leaks.

During the catheter insertion procedure, the access provider should attach devices for catheter adaptation and transfer/extension. If the catheter gets contaminated, the transfer set and the lower portion of the catheter can be removed and replaced. This will spare the nursing staff to go through the replacement of the entire catheter. The transfer/extension set should be separate from the surgical dressing, allowing the nursing staff access to flushing without excessive manipulation of the dressing.

The experienced nursing staff applies the surgical dressing, which immobilizes the catheter and prevents contamination of the exit site and possible trauma. The most used dressings are the nonocclusive gauze dressings. They allow the drainage to be away from the insertion and the exit sites. Changing the dressing should be done after 5–10 days, except in cases where bleeding or infection occurs. Postoperative dressing changes should be done only by experienced nurses. If the patient lives far from the center, the nurses should be properly trained before allowing the patient to change the dressing. Patients are not allowed to shower until the nursing staff determines that it is safe to do so. This is done to prevent contamination and infection of the healing exit site. The patient should be instructed to avoid moving the catheter excessively because this may increase the risk of infection. The patient should be educated to call the nursing team if they notice signs of infection or if injury to the catheter occurs.

The most common complications of peritoneal catheters are infectious and mechanical. With proper catheter placement and care, the chances of these complications are minimal, and the catheter will continue to work for many years.

Exchange Procedures and Sterile Techniques

During the exchange procedure, a type of solution called dialysate is instilled into the peritoneal cavity through an appropriately placed peritoneal catheter. The average volume of solution used in adults is two liters. Lower volumes are used in children or smaller patients, and higher volumes are used in large patients.

The fluid dwells in the abdominal cavity for a defined period called the dwell period. The dwell period varies in length in different PD techniques. During the dwell period, processes such as solute diffusion and ultrafiltration occur. These processes are bidirectional. When the dialysate and the peritoneal capillaries come into contact, urea, potassium, and creatinine diffuse from the blood into the dialysate. In peritoneal dialysis, glucose in the dialysate acts as an osmotic agent to facilitate ultrafiltration. The speed of the solute transport depends on the peritoneal vascularity. When the exchange procedure ends, the used dialysate is discarded. The cycle then gets repeated.

Continuous Ambulatory Peritoneal Dialysis (CAPD) Technique

In CAPD, after the dialysate dwells in the peritoneal cavity, it is drained out into a separate drainage bag, not back into the same bag that was used for filling. Each exchange involves using a fresh bag of dialysate for filling, and the waste dialysate is drained into a separate empty bag. This process reduces the risk of infection and ensures the effectiveness of the dialysis. The patient or caregiver performs four to five exchanges manually during the day and one during the night. The day dwell time usually lasts from 4–6 hours each, whereas the night dwell lasts approximately 8–9 hours. The exchanges can be done at any clean, dry place, and the patient is allowed to proceed with their regular activities during the process.

Automated Peritoneal Dialysis (APD) Technique

APD treatment frees up more time during the day compared to CAPD, which makes it more convenient for most patients and their caregivers. APD regimens are divided into four different types:

Continuous cycling peritoneal dialysis (CCPD) – it consists of 4–5 nighttime exchanges over 9–10 hours, and a final exchange with a long daytime dwell. This regimen is the one that is most commonly used.

Nightly intermittent peritoneal dialysis (NIPD) – it consists of 4–5-night exchanges and no fluid in the peritoneal cavity during the day.

Classical intermittent peritoneal dialysis (CIPD) – This method consists of APD treatments several times a week. It has been avoided due to poor clearances and high morbidity and mortality rates.

Tidal peritoneal dialysis (TPD) – This method is rarely used.

Aseptic Precautions

Nurses are expected to follow sterile techniques during the catheter placement and exchange procedures. Patients should be educated on aseptic practices such as hand hygiene, use of masks, and maintenance of a safe environment where exchanges can be carried out. The patients, family members, and the healthcare team are expected to have excellent hand hygiene before starting the exchange procedure. The most preferred method is to rub the hands with 70% alcohol solution for at least 15 seconds. Hand cleansing is done by handwashing for 15 seconds with antimicrobial soap (4% chlorhexidine). If the hands are visibly dirty, they should be washed with soap. Multiple-dose vials such as heparin or potassium chloride should not be used as dialysate supplements because they increase the risk of introducing microorganisms during the injection. Chlorhexidine and alcohol should be scrubbed on the injection ports. Patients should be instructed to apply topical antibiotics such as mupirocin or gentamicin cream or ointment on the existing site. This should be done daily. The area where the dialysis procedures will be performed should always be kept clean, well-lit, dry, and pet-free.

Chapter 18: Complications and Management in Peritoneal Dialysis

Infectious Complications

Peritonitis

Peritonitis is a common complication among patients who undergo peritoneal dialysis (PD). The incidence of peritonitis is dependent on several factors. Factors include age, patient wellbeing, and PD modality. The risk of peritonitis in PD patients is influenced by several factors including the patient's technique, adherence to aseptic procedures, and individual circumstances. By far, the most common pathogens responsible for peritonitis are gram-positive organisms. Most cases of PD-associated peritonitis are caused by gram-positive pathogens, whereas a third of cases result from gram-negative bacteria. In 20% of cases, the cultures return negative. This distribution changes slightly with age. The Korean pediatric report states that the majority of peritonitis in pediatric patients is precipitated by gram-positive bacteria. Fungi are responsible for only a fraction of peritonitis cases, according to the SCOPE report. These pathogens mostly affect children under the age of 2 years old. Fungal peritonitis in children is associated with a higher risk of hospital admission, longer hospital stays, and an elevated rate of technique failure.

The diagnosis of peritonitis is confirmed by analyzing effluent peritoneal fluid, which tends to be cloudy due to the increased leukocyte count. Microbial studies include cell count, differential count, and culture. If white blood cells (WBCs) exceed 100/mm^3, with a minimal 50% of WBCs as polymorphonuclear leukocytes, the diagnosis of peritonitis is confirmed.

To manage PD-associated peritonitis, antibiotics should be administered through the intraperitoneal route. Research advocates for the continuous administration of beta-lactam antibiotics. The exchange with the loading dose remains for 4–6 hours, whereas the subsequent exchanges for the remaining treatment course should contain the maintenance dose.

Patients who receive intermittent therapy should get the dose once a day in the long dwell. Extending the dwell time to 3–6 hours is necessary for patients on nocturnal automated peritoneal dialysis with short dwell times.

The recommended empiric antibiotic to treat peritonitis is vancomycin or first-generation cephalosporin combined with an aminoglycoside or a third-generation cephalosporin. There is some evidence that cefepime can be used as monotherapy due to its significant activity against gram-positive and gram-negative bacteria.

When the culture results are ready, healthcare practitioners should tailor the antibiotics accordingly. For instance, if the culture reveals gram-positive bacteria that are sensitive to first-generation cephalosporins, it's important to discontinue aminoglycosides and third-generation cephalosporins. The combination of a first-generation cephalosporin with a glycopeptide, such as vancomycin, is advised in patients who have a history of MRSA infection or when the center-specific resistance rate of MRSA is greater than 10%. Patients with a documented allergy to beta-lactams (e.g., penicillins, cephalosporins) can also receive a glycopeptide. It is important to monitor the blood levels of antibiotics in patients treated with intermittent doses of glycopeptides.

Additional recommendations by the International Society of Peritoneal Dialysis (ISPD) include adding rifampin in patients with a delayed response to therapy with a positive culture for *Staphylococcus aureus* and coagulase-negative *Staphylococcus aureus*. The duration of treatment ranges between 2–3 weeks for positive cultures, with *Staphylococcus aureus* and enterococci. Coagulase-negative *Staphylococcus* requires 21 days of antibiotics. Streptococcus-triggered peritonitis should last at least 14 days.

For non-*Pseudomonas*, gram-negative bacteria, ceftazidime or cefepime are recommended as first-line agents. When *Pseudomonas* species is cultured, it is recommended to add another antibiotic agent that's effective against this bacterium but exerts a different action mechanism. The treatment duration for gram-negative bacteria ranges between 3–4 weeks, whereas *Pseudomonas*-triggered peritonitis should receive at least 21 days of antibiotics.

In a subset of patients, the cultures will come back negative after 72 hours despite the highly suspicious clinical presentation of peritonitis. In this case, empiric antibiotics (e.g., cefepime, cefazoline, ceftazidime, glycopeptide) should be continued for two weeks.

Finally, PD catheter removal is recommended in patients with refractory bacterial peritonitis, exit-site infections, fungal peritonitis, and tunnel infections with the same bacteria.

Exit-site Infections

Exit-site infection (ESI) is a relatively common complication of peritoneal dialysis seen in 0.25 per dialysis year. The risk of ESI varies based on multiple factors, including the patient's overall health, hygiene practices, and catheter care techniques, rather than age alone. The culprit agent for ESI is predominantly bacteria, including *Staphylococcus aureus* or *Staphylococcus epidermidis*. These microbes come in contact with the exit site during catheter care, which can develop due to unsterile catheters or contaminated hands. Healthcare professionals should pay attention to the risk factors of ESI, such as obesity, diabetes, immunosuppression, and a history of previous ESIs.

The cardinal signs and symptoms of an ESI include erythema, edema, tenderness, pain, and purulent discharge at the catheter exit site. Patients may also present with generalized symptoms, such as fever, lethargy, and general malaise.

To evaluate the status of the exit site during peritoneal dialysis, healthcare providers rely on a scoring system that also considers edema at the exit site, erythema, pain, crust, and secretions (see table 8).

Table 8: Criteria to Diagnose Exit-site Infections

Exit-site Score			
	0	1	2
Pain on pressure	No	Exit site (<0.5 cm)	More parts of the tunnel
Crust	No	<0.5 cm	>0.5 cm
Redness	No	<0.5 cm	>0.5 cm
Swelling	No	Slight	Large
Secretion	No	Serous	Purulent

A score above 4 should prompt the diagnosis of ESI. Uncomplicated ESI can be treated with oral antibiotics for at least 2 weeks. Patients should keep taking oral antibiotics for 7 days after the resolution of infection signs. The duration of treatment is prolonged to 3 weeks in patients with confirmed *Staphylococcus aureus* or *Pseudomonas* infections.

Catheter immobilization can help lower the incidence of ESI. In cases where chronic exit site care is required, daily application of topical antibiotics (e.g., gentamicin) and cleansing of the site with a sterile antiseptic/gauze is necessary.

Tunnel Infections

Tunnel infections describe the spread of microbial agents into the catheter tunnel. Some healthcare professionals think of tunnel infections as a complication of exit-site infection. Similar to ESI, the main microbes that cause tunnel infections include *Staphylococcus aureus* and *Staphylococcus epidermidis*. Studies objectified a few risk factors, including poor hygiene during catheter care, obesity, diabetes, and immunosuppression.

Patients will report tenderness and pain along the tunnel path, as well as a general feeling of unwellness. Objective findings include fever, erythema, edema, and purulent discharges.

The management of tunnel infections is mainly dependent on the level of infection and involvement of the deep cuff. To investigate this finding, it's important to assess the presence of fluids around the superficial cuff. The absence of fluids implies that the infection is restricted to the exit site.

Ultrasound may be useful when assessing fluids around the superficial cuff and is sufficient to diagnose catheter tunnel infection even in the absence of deep cuff involvement or concurrent peritonitis.

A more sophisticated approach to manage tunnel infections includes the conservative excision of exit site skin over to the subcutaneous track until the superficial cuff is visible. Subsequently, the cuff is shaved and the catheter is immobilized. Alternatively, the exit site and the skin that covers the subcutaneous track is excised, along with the tissue around the catheter segment that contains the superficial cuff.

In practice, the vast majority of tunnel infection cases are addressed by the removal of the old catheter and the insertion of a new one in a different site. If the microbes reach the deep cuff and cause peritonitis, healthcare professionals should follow the steps covered in the previous section.

Mechanical Complications

Impaired Catheter Flow

Catheter flow may be impaired during dialysate infusion or drainage of the peritoneal cavity. The incidence of catheter flow issues varies significantly from one source to another. To reduce this risk, laparoscopic techniques are the ideal choice to insert the catheter. Impaired flow may be due to catheter malposition, catheter kinking, catheter entrapment, and extra/intraluminal catheter occlusions.

Depending on the etiology, the timing of impaired catheter flow will be different. Generally, catheter malposition, kinking, and entrapment occur during the first month of catheter use. Catheter malposition is usually a more common cause of flow problems, which occur when the catheter tip is not properly placed in the pelvis. Also, catheter kinking is a possible complication. Conversely, intraluminal and extraluminal catheter occlusion may occur later in the process. The pathophysiology revolves around the formation of a fibrin clot, which explains the delayed onset of these flow issues.

Some clinicians may choose to categorize flow problems into outflow and inflow issues. Impairment could also be a bidirectional obstruction, which blocks the inflow and outflow of dialysate. Causes of outflow obstruction are usually extraluminal catheter occlusion, catheter entrapment, and catheter malposition. Bidirectional obstruction is commonly seen in intraluminal catheter occlusion and catheter kinking.

One clinical feature of outflow obstruction is pain with dialysate drainage. However, this is neither sensitive nor specific.

Management of impaired catheter flow includes flushing the catheter with saline or heparin to clear the obstruction. Moreover, it's useful to adjust and reposition the catheter to ensure it is not kinked or twisted. Significant catheter exchange may be warranted in severe obstructions.

To prevent impaired catheter flow, close attention should be paid to proper catheter placement, securing techniques, and regular catheter care. Adequate flushing of the catheter with sterile saline or heparin solution can help prevent clot formation.

Regular follow-up is important to monitor catheter function and address any issues promptly. Patients should be educated to recognize and report symptoms of impaired catheter flow.

Fluid Leaks

Dialysate fluid leaks are from the potential complications of peritoneal dialysis. The most common among the leaks is the pericatheter leak. It's also possible for fluid leaks to occur in other areas, such as the trocaremployed site, extra-abdominal leaks (e.g., hydrothorax, pericardial effusion), and inguinal site, which presents as genital edema.

Some risk factors for dialysate fluid leaks include catheter malposition, increased intra-abdominal pressure due to coughing, sneezing, bowel movement straining, catheter-related infections, and dialysate issues (e.g., too warm or too cold).

Signs and symptoms of fluid leaks include fluid drainage/dampness, discomfort, and pigmentation changes in the skin around the exit site.

Preventive measures focus on the proper insertion and positioning of the catheter, proper hygiene, the temperature of the dialysate, and activities that increase intra-abdominal pressure.

The management of fluid leaks serves to lower the dialysate volume with a cycler to perform PD and switch to hemodialysis (combined with surgical repair).

Hernias

Increased intra-abdominal pressure after the insertion of the catheter may precipitate hernia. Risk factors for this mechanical complication include multiparity, malnutrition, immunosuppression, and weak anterior muscles of the abdomen.

Types of hernias are exit-site hernias, peristomal hernias, and incisional hernias. Patients will commonly report discomfort, irregular bowel movement, and a visible bulge in the anterior abdomen.

Risk factors play a vital role in the development of hernias during peritoneal dialysis. Multiparity can weaken the abdominal muscles and increase the risk of herniation. Malnutrition is another contributing factor, as it causes muscle weakness and decreases tissue integrity. Patients who receive immunosuppressive therapy in the context of organ transplantation are also at a higher risk of developing PD-associated hernias. Additionally, individuals with weak anterior abdominal muscles are prone to develop this mechanical complication.

Several measures can lower the risk of hernias associated with peritoneal dialysis. This includes education on lifting techniques and activities that reduce intra-abdominal pressure, proper catheter placement, and monitoring of the signs of hernia during routine care.

The management of hernia can be conservative or surgical. Conservative management includes supportive garments to dampen the strain, whereas surgical intervention focuses on closing the defect and reinforcement of the anterior abdominal wall.

Hydrothorax

Hydrothorax in peritoneal dialysis describes the accumulation of dialysate in the pleural space. Although this complication only affects a few patients, it can be life-threatening. Patients with hydrothorax normally present with symptoms of hydrothorax, such as dyspnea and acute transudative pleural effusion, within the first 30 days of initiating dialysis. The pathogenesis of hydrothorax in this context is catheter dysfunction or increased peritoneal pressure.

The main cause of hydrothorax in PD patients is pleuroperitoneal communication, which is associated with congenital or acquired defects in the diaphragm. Moreover, malpositioned or malfunctioning catheters can also contribute to hydrothorax. Interestingly, hydrothorax is predominantly observed on the right side due to partial support of the left diaphragm by the heart and the pericardium. Patients may experience crushing chest pain, dyspnea, and cough during dialysate indwelling, albeit some patients are asymptomatic or exhibit mild symptoms.

The prognosis for patients with hydrothorax depends on timely diagnosis, the effectiveness of the chosen treatment approach, and the patient's overall health status. Imaging tests (e.g., chest CT, X-ray imaging, ultrasonography) can confirm the presence of pleural fluid but may not reveal the underlying diaphragmatic defect. Elevated glucose levels in the pleural fluid suggest pleuroperitoneal communication but are not universally reliable. Today, peritoneal scintigraphy is the imaging modality of choice to diagnose hydrothorax and identify diaphragmatic defects.

The management of hydrothorax centers around the discontinuation of PD for 4–6 weeks and the transition to hemodialysis. This approach allows the mediastinum to heal and prevents further effusions. About one quarter of patients respond positively to this treatment. More invasive options include hemodialysis and invasive procedures to continue PD. These invasive measures are mechanical pleurodesis via abrasive pad placement during open or video thoracotomy and chemical pleurodesis that uses agents, such as povidone, talc, or tetracycline through catheter infusion. Pleurodesis reduces the risk of hydrothorax for up to 50 months post-treatment.

In cases with significant defects, video-assisted thoracoscopic repair or thoracotomy and direct vision repair are performed. Some innovative techniques involve the use of automatic endoscopic staplers, endoscopic suturing devices, nonabsorbable mesh, and fibrin glue to close diaphragmatic defects. After the intervention, it is common to discontinue PD for several weeks to allow the diaphragm to heal.

Despite the vagueness of the long-term success of these procedures, patients who experience hydrothorax early in their PD treatment often return to PD as their preferred dialysis method. However, for patients who cannot or do not wish to undergo invasive procedures, it's essential to switch to hemodialysis.

Metabolic and Physiologic Complications

Protein Loss

Protein loss is a prominent complication during peritoneal dialysis, especially when associated with peritonitis. Estimates place the rate of protein loss at 0.5 g/L to 4 g/L during intermittent PD. The usual amount of protein lost in peritoneal dialysis ranges from 5 to 15 grams per day. Stable patients on continuous ambulatory peritoneal dialysis are estimated to lose around 5 g of protein per day. The rate of protein loss worsens in patients with acute kidney injury and/or high-volume peritoneal dialysis (HVPD) combined with peritonitis or ascites.

The pathophysiology of protein loss during peritoneal dialysis revolves around increased peritoneal membrane permeability, the choice of dialysate solution (i.e., high glucose concentration may increase protein loss), low-grade inflammation within the peritoneal cavity, and genetics (e.g., high peritoneal transporters).

The clinical manifestations resemble signs and symptoms of malnutrition, such as unintentional weight loss, muscle wasting, and edema. However, the prevalence of these symptoms varies significantly from one patient to another.

Monitoring patients who exhibit signs of protein loss is indispensable. Healthcare providers should pay close attention to the clinical signs of malnutrition and fluid overload, as well as run frequent serum protein levels and protein concentrations in the dialysate effluent.

The management of protein loss in PD requires specialists to modify the composition of the dialysate (e.g., lower glucose concentrations), adjust dialysis (e.g., dwell time), provide nutritional support, and address subsequent complications (e.g., inflammation, infection).

Hyperglycemia

Hyperglycemia in the context of peritoneal dialysis is another common metabolic complication that requires deep understanding to manage it. Serum tonicity mainly depends on serum glucose and sodium. Hyperglycemia in peritoneal dialysis patients, results from the high glucose content in the dialysate, and can cause increased serum tonicity.

Clinicians need to categorize hyperglycemia in PD patients based on renal function to tailor the management approach.

Patients with Preserved Renal Function

In this group of patients, hyperglycemia leads to hypertonicity due to high glucose levels in the serum combined with hypotonic fluid loss through osmotic diuresis.

Oligo-anuric Patients

Oligo-anuric patients experience more modest hypertonicity during hyperglycemia. This is mostly due to high levels of glucose without significant hypotonic fluid loss. However, some factors, such as thirst regulation and water intake, can influence hypertonicity in these patients.

Sodium Levels in Hyperglycemia

Hypertonicity caused by isolated hyperglycemia may lead to hyponatremia. This phenomenon occurs because intracellular water exits into the extracellular compartment and dilutes sodium levels. Hyperglycemic hypertonicity can mask this decrease in serum sodium concentration.

Severe hypertonicity observed in some PD patients may be attributed to the following factors:

Prolonged Peritoneal Dialysis

The use of hypertonic dialysate during peritoneal dialysis, especially with short dwell times, can contribute to excessive hypertonicity due to water loss through peritoneal ultrafiltration.

Anasarca

The presence of anasarca (i.e., generalized swelling) can exacerbate hypertonicity. Anasarca significantly affects the levels of serum sodium and tonicity during treatment.

A key factor that modifies tonicity during hyperglycemia correction is the expansion of extracellular volume. Patients with significant hyperglycemia and increased extracellular volume experience slower decreases in serum sodium concentration and faster increases in tonicity. This relationship highlights the interaction between extracellular volume and tonicity fluctuations.

Potassium Levels and Hyperglycemia

Another aspect to consider is the hypokalemia associated with hyperglycemia treated with insulin in oligo-anuric patients. In some cases, serum potassium levels may remain unchanged due to numerous factors, such as extracellular volume contraction or ongoing catabolism.

Acid-based Disturbances and Hyperglycemia

In patients with hyperglycemia, the more common acid-base disturbance is metabolic acidosis. This phenomenon highlights why acid-base disturbances should be monitored and managed during hyperglycemia treatment in PD patients.

Fluid Imbalances

Healthcare providers often face difficulties when assessing the volume status of patients on PD. Conventionally, clinical evaluation has been the primary method to determine volume status in PD patients. Despite integrating advanced technologies, such as bioimpedance analysis and lung ultrasound, in volume status assessment, the research could not objectify the superiority of these methods over conventional clinical evaluation. Therefore, it is recommended to use these technologies as adjuncts to clinical evaluation rather than standalone methods to assess fluid imbalances in PD.

Despite the lack of consensus when defining volume overload in PD, healthcare providers should pay attention to the following symptoms: gradual weight gain, elevated blood pressure, elevated jugular venous pressure, and inspiratory crackles. The absence of edema does not necessarily rule out fluid overload, especially in younger patients. Conversely, peripheral edema may be present but not always associated with true volume overload, as it can occur in patients who take certain medications or those with hypoalbuminemia.

The incidence of volume overload in patients who undergo peritoneal dialysis can vary. There is also an objective increase in the risk of cardiovascular mortality. Untreated volume overload can lead to technique failure in PD and a premature transition to hemodialysis (HD).

The risk factors of volume overload in PD include increased dietary salt intake, drinking too much fluids, reduced residual kidney function, and inadequate peritoneal ultrafiltration (the process of removing excess fluid from the peritoneal cavity). Clinicians should consider these factors when addressing volume overload to identify reversible risk factors.

Managing volume overload in PD starts with patient education to lower salt and fluid intake. For patients with residual kidney function, high doses of diuretics (e.g., furosemide, metolazone, spironolactone) can be considered as well. Additionally, it may be effective to adjust PD to maximize the osmotic pressure and fluid removal. Unfortunately, this approach may have limitations due to the risk of prolonged glucose exposure.

In cases of acute symptomatic volume overload in PD, healthcare providers should attempt to use hypertonic solutions and high-dose diuretics to maximize PD ultrafiltration before the transition to hemodialysis. Transition to hemodialysis should only be suggested for patients with refractory hypervolemia.

Chapter 19: Transplant and Acute Therapies

Adequate acute care for a renal transplant patient is vital to support transplant function, aid in rapid recovery, and ensure the long-term success of the transplant. The acute therapy protocol for kidney transplant patients prioritizes patient stabilization and proper fluid-electrolyte balance. It also includes the administration of immunosuppressive drugs. Furthermore, health professionals strive to promptly monitor and address complications while continuously evaluating the graft function.

Immediate Postoperative Care

Vital Sign Monitoring and Stabilization

Patients' vital signs should be monitored every 30 minutes until they stabilize and then hourly for the next 12 hours, every 2 hours for the next 8 hours, and then every 4 hours. Continuous ECG monitoring is an option for high-risk patients.

Respiratory depression in the immediate postoperative period for kidney transplant patients is typically related to residual effects of anesthetic agents and pain medications. Chest physiotherapy and incentive spirometry can be used every hour to improve respiratory function.

The patient is encouraged to ambulate early, usually on the first postoperative day. Feeding is usually started on the first postoperative day with clear fluids.

Maintaining Fluid and Electrolyte Balance

Post-transplant patients could have a high urine output secondary to osmotic diuresis. This may result from intraoperative administration of furosemide, excessive intraoperative IV fluid administration, or preoperative fluid overload. Thus, fluid intake and output should be monitored hourly using urine output and central venous pressure (CVP). Since it increases renal blood flow and diuresis, dopamine should be discontinued if used intraoperatively. In addition to urine output, weight should also be measured daily.

Correct the fluid balance based on the urine output and CVP. Target a CVP of 10–15 cm H_2O and an hourly urine output of at least 0.5 ml/kg/hr.

The choice of maintenance fluid is 5% dextrose with half-strength NS. The only exceptions are diabetic patients who should use the half-strength NS alone. The daily maintenance fluid is around 1500 cc per 24 hours. The table below shows that the amount of replacement fluid administered depends on the patient's urine output.

Table 9: Maintenance and Replacement Fluid Therapy for Transplant Patients

Urine output:	The amount of maintenance and replacement fluid that should be administered:
≤200 ml/hr.	Replace ml for ml.
>200 ml/hr.	200 ml + 0.5 ml for each ml above 200.
>300 ml/hr for four consecutive hours or >500 ml/hr for two consecutive hours.	Hold replacement fluid and reassess after 2 hours.

If the urine output is <50 ml/hr or if there is an abrupt cessation of urine output, the patency of the catheter should be checked. If the anuria persists, imaging studies like Doppler ultrasound and radioisotope scan should be done to evaluate the blood flow to the transplanted kidney.

Postoperative electrolyte abnormalities are common. Thus, the serum electrolyte level should be monitored every 6 hours for the first three days and daily afterward. SGOT, SGPT, LDH, ALP, and total bilirubin should be done twice a week.

Pain Management

Pain management reduces anxiety, facilitates deep breathing and early ambulation, and improves patient satisfaction. The most commonly used class of analgesics is opiates. Pethidine should be avoided because its metabolites could accumulate due to reduced renal function.

Wound Management

Since immunosuppressive drugs impair wound healing, adequate wound care is necessary to facilitate wound healing. Wound care should be carried out daily and on a PRN basis. Abdominal drainage may be inserted during the operation, and it should be removed when drainage output is <50 ml for at least two consecutive days. This usually occurs on days 5 to 6.

Catheter Care

A catheter is left in place after surgery, and the drainage may be bloody due to the surgical procedure. If the hematuria is severe, clots could form, which could result in anuria and suprapubic pain. Bladder irrigation can be done in these cases.

Urine output should be recorded every 24 hours, and samples should be collected for urinalysis, culture, and sensitivity. The routine for catheter care and removal can vary based on the patient's condition and the specific protocols of the healthcare facility.

Immunosuppressive Therapy

Immunosuppressive therapy is initiated at or before kidney transplantation. It has 3 phases: induction, initial maintenance, and long-term maintenance. Interleukin-2 receptor antagonists are first-line drugs for the induction phase, followed by lymphocyte-depleting agents. In the initial maintenance phase, patients are started on a calcineurin inhibitor (cyclosporin or tacrolimus) and an antiproliferative agent (mycophenolate mofetil). After 2-4 months, treatment is continued with the lowest calcineurin inhibitor dose. During treatment, calcineurin inhibitor levels should be monitored daily until the target level is reached. CNI levels should also be monitored when there is a decline in kidney function or a change in patient status.

Early Surgical Complications

Urinary Tract Complications

Urinary Obstruction

Urinary obstruction should be considered in a patient with a decreased urine output who is not responding to a fluid challenge. It could be from catheter obstruction, bladder dysfunction, or ureteral obstruction. Thus, the first step is to check whether or not the catheter is patent and functioning correctly by irrigating it. Next to catheter malfunction, the second most common cause of urinary obstruction is bladder dysfunction. A trial of alpha-blockers like prazosin can be used to check for this condition. If the bladder is still dysfunctional after one to two trials of alpha-blockers, intermittent catheterization may be necessary. An abdominal ultrasound can be done to check for ureteral obstruction. If the bladder is collapsed and there is pelvicaliceal dilation, it implies ureteral obstruction. The best treatment option in this case would be urgent decompression with a nephrostomy tube.

Urine Leak

Postoperative urine leak is usually due to a surgical problem with ureteroneocystostomy or ischemic necrosis of the distal ureter. Patients present with abdominal pain, decreased urine output, and increased serum creatinine. Urinoma (i.e., urine collection around the kidney and the bladder) could also manifest with pain and swelling at the incision site. The collection can be confirmed with an abdominal ultrasound. Immediate surgical correction is necessary.

Vascular Complications

Arterial Stenosis

Transplant artery stenosis may manifest with fluid retention, hypertension, and rising serum creatinine. Cyclosporine and tacrolimus are both calcineurin inhibitors used in transplant immunosuppression, and they have been associated with nephrotoxicity. Magnetic resonance angiography is the investigation of choice for patients suspected of this condition. It can be treated with either balloon dilation or surgery.

Renal Vein Thrombosis

Renal vein thrombosis occurs when the renal vein has been narrowed by repair of an injury, when the vein was twisted, or when it is compressed externally. Patients manifest with the sudden onset of gross hematuria, anuria, and pain and swelling at the incision site. Renal Doppler ultrasound shows absent flow in the renal vein and reversed diastolic flow in the renal artery. An immediate surgical repair should be carried out.

Postoperative Bleeding

Postoperative bleeding usually emerges within 24-48 hours post-surgery. It is characterized by a decrease in hematocrit, a bulge at the incision site, or blood seepage from the incision site. It is common in patients who take anticoagulant medication for a different medical reason. Imaging with ultrasound or a CT scan should be done to evaluate the extent of hematoma if it is not clinically apparent. Treatment could range from a blood transfusion to immediate surgery.

Early Medical Complications

Common Post-transplant Infections

Even though kidney transplantation is associated with a lower risk of infection than other solid organ transplantations, infection is the second most common cause of death in renal transplant patients after cardiovascular disease. The typical infection etiologies, in decreasing frequency, are viruses, gram-positive bacteria, gram-negative bacteria, mycobacterial infections, fungal infections, and parasitic infections.

Viral Infections

Viral infections are the most common infection in renal transplant patients, especially during the first six months. The commonly identified viruses are CMV, HSV, HBV, HCV, human polyomavirus, and EBV.

Cytomegalovirus (CMV)

Without antiviral prophylaxis, symptomatic CMV occurs in 6% of transplant patients. Patients might be infected in one of the following three ways:

- Primary infection: Previously uninfected, seronegative patients contract the infection either via blood transfusion or from the donated organ. Only 40-50% of these patients are symptomatic.
- Reactivation: The virus gets reactivated and causes infection in previously seropositive patients. 10-15% of patients on immunosuppressive therapy develop symptomatic CMV infection.
- Superinfection: CMV superinfection usually refers to a scenario where a CMV-seropositive recipient (a person who already has CMV antibodies) receives an organ from a CMV-seropositive donor and subsequently develops an active CMV infection.

Patients with CMV infection usually become symptomatic 4-8 weeks after transplantation. It can manifest as a non-specific febrile syndrome with neutropenia or cause a direct tissue-invasive disease like pneumonia, hepatitis, pancreatitis, or GI invasion.

The gold standard for diagnosis is demonstrating the inclusion of bodies in tissues. DNA PCR can also be used for diagnosis and treatment response monitoring. Although serologic studies can help predict risk before transplantation, they are less helpful in defining clinical disease since they cannot differentiate active from passive infection.

CMV prophylaxis is recommended for the first three months after transplant and the first six weeks after T–cell depleting antibody therapy unless both the donor and the recipient are seronegative for CMV. The agents of choice are oral ganciclovir or oral valganciclovir. These agents can also be used to treat patients with mild clinical symptoms. Patients with tissue-invasive CMV infections should be treated with IV ganciclovir. Patients with active disease should be monitored weekly using Nucleic Acid Amplification testing (NAT), such as DNA or PCR. Treatment should be continued until the virus is undetectable.

HSV and VZV

The frequency of HSV reactivation and invasive HSV infection is increased in transplant patients, with most cases occurring during the first month after transplantation. A superficial HSV infection should be treated with oral acyclovir, famciclovir, or valacyclovir until no new active lesions are present. This reduces dissemination. In the case of systemic HSV infection, immunosuppressive drugs should be withdrawn and treated with IV acyclovir for 14-21 days. Prophylactic therapy for HSV infection is recommended for patients who have frequent recurrences.

Transplant patients are treated with primary varicella zoster infection with oral acyclovir 80 mg/kg/day in 4 divided doses for seven days. Uncomplicated herpes zoster is treated with oral acyclovir until all the lesions have scabbed. If herpes zoster involves more than three dermatomes, it is called invasive zoster, and it should be treated with IV acyclovir and immunosuppressive medications should be withdrawn. Varicella immunoglobulin can be given to transplant patients exposed to varicella infection within 96 hours. If it is unavailable or has been more than 96 hours, prophylaxis is provided with a 7-day course of oral acyclovir.

HCV and HBV

Renal transplant patients who are positive for HBsAg (Hepatitis B surface antigen) should receive antiviral prophylaxis. Interferon is generally avoided in transplant patients due to its immunomodulatory effects, which can potentially increase the risk of graft rejection.

For patients with HCV, the benefit of treatment should outweigh the risk of graft rejection secondary to interferon-based therapy. If the benefit outweighs the risk and treatment is started, HCV RNA level, ALT, and a test for proteinuria should be done every 3-6 months. If the protein-to-creatinine ratio is >1 or the 24-hour urine protein is >1 gram on at least two occasions, further investigation with a graft biopsy is needed to assess graft dysfunction.

In the early postoperative period, the common bacterial pathogens are MRSA, pseudomonas species, and Enterobacteriaceae like E. coli and Klebsiella.

UTI

The most common bacterial infection seen in renal transplant patients is urinary tract infection (UTI). A UTI could be severe enough to cause graft failure, sepsis, and death. The risk of UTI is highest during the first six post-transplant months. Thus, we administer a prophylactic antibiotic during this period. Even though ciprofloxacin effectively prevents UTIs, it has been associated with an increased risk of pneumocystis jirovecii (PCP) pneumonia. Hence, trimethoprim-sulfamethoxazole (TMP-SMX) is our drug of choice for prophylaxis. If the patient is allergic to TMP-SMX, we can use nitrofurantoin. Patients with allograft-associated pyelonephritis should be admitted to the hospital and treated with IV antibiotics.

Tuberculosis

The incidence of active tuberculosis in renal transplant patients is estimated to be 1 to 4 percent. The most frequent source of infection is the reactivation of latent TB. Approximately 40% of transplant patients with active TB develop disseminated infections involving the skin, skeletal system, and CNS. The standard treatment regimen for active tuberculosis generally involves a two-month initial phase of rifampin, isoniazid, pyrazinamide, and ethambutol, followed by a continuation phase of four months of rifampin and isoniazid.

Prophylactic treatment should be administered to patients with evidence of a latent TB infection. Tuberculin skin tests or interferon-gamma assays can be used to diagnose latent TB. A 9-month course of prophylactic isoniazid can be administered for patients proven to have latent TB using either of these methods, regardless of BCG vaccination status.

Both isoniazid and rifampin have effects on the cytochrome p-450 enzyme system. Isoniazid increases the level of mTOR and calcineurin inhibitors, and rifampicin decreases the level of these drugs. These drug interactions increase the risk of graft rejection. We can use rifabutin instead of rifampicin since it is not a strong inducer of CYP3A4.

Fungal Infections

Candida is the most common fungal pathogen in renal transplant patients, with most infections occurring in the first postoperative month. Candida albicans is the most common species, followed by Candida glabrata, Candida tropicalis, and Candida parapsilosis. Mucocutaneous infection is the most common. In addition to this, it could also infect wounds, cause intra-abdominal infections, and complicate viral infections (HSV, VZV). Prophylaxis with oral clotrimazole, nystatin, or oral fluconazole should be provided for 1-3 months and one month after treatment with anti-lymphocyte antibody therapy.

Vaccination

The influenza vaccine is not a live vaccine. It is an inactivated vaccine and is recommended for renal transplant patients, including during the first six months after transplantation. Other than that, the vaccines recommended for renal transplant patients are the same as the general population. Since there is intense immune suppression during the first 3-6 months, vaccine administration should be avoided. However, influenza virus can be administered as early as one month. Anti-HBS antibody titers should guide HBV vaccine administration. Antibody titers should be determined 6-12 weeks after HBV vaccination completion. Revaccination is indicated if the titer is <10 mIU/ml.

Post-transplant Hypertension

The prevalence of hypertension in patients with renal transplants is between 60-80%. Even though the exact pathogenesis is unknown, factors like immunosuppressive medications and renal artery stenosis have been implicated. Steroids can mediate salt and water retention, decrease prostaglandin synthesis, and increase the smooth vessel pressure response. Calcineurin inhibitors elevate blood pressure through sodium and water retention enhancement, sympathetic nervous system activity augmentation, and intra-renal renin biosynthesis upregulation. Post-transplant hypertension is associated with chronic graft nephropathy, rejection, and increased mortality.

Many antihypertensive drugs treat post-transplant hypertension. Nevertheless, ARBs or ACE inhibitors are the first lines in patients with proteinuria >1 gram per 24 hours. The blood pressure target should be <130/80 mmHg.

Graft Function

Assessing Graft Function

Graft function is assessed using serum creatinine, urine protein excretion, and urine output.

Monitor serum creatinine levels daily during the initial week, followed by a frequency of every 2 to 3 days over the subsequent 2-4 weeks. Then, transition to a weekly monitoring regimen lasting 2 to 3 months. After this period, adjust to bi-weekly checks for the next 4 to 6 months, and finally, proceed with monthly assessments from the seventh until the twelfth month. Urine protein excretion should be measured once in the first month to establish a baseline and every three months for the first year. Urine output should be measured every hour until graft function is stable.

Patients with immediate graft function have adequate urine output and a decrease in serum creatinine by 1 to >4 mg/dl daily. Patients with slowly recovering graft function are non-oliguric, and the creatinine level decreases by 0.2 mg/dl daily. These patients do not require dialysis unless it is complicated by fluid overload, hyperkalemia, or severe anemia requiring blood transfusion. Patients with delayed graft function are oliguric and require support with dialysis for volume, hyperkalemia, or uremia.

Graft Rejection

Hyperacute Rejection

This occurs in patients with an ABO mismatch or a positive lymphocytotoxic cross-match. In hyperacute rejection, patients are anuric, and the kidney does not have blood flow on Doppler ultrasound because of microvascular thrombosis. The treatment is immediate surgery.

Acute Rejection

This is the most common form of rejection. It usually occurs 5 to 7 days post-transplant and is caused by T-lymphocyte-mediated allograft injury. Patients present with fever, an increasing creatinine level, weight gain, and graft tenderness. Patients taking tacrolimus and cyclosporine seldom present with fever and tenderness. A kidney biopsy should be done to confirm the diagnosis if acute rejection is suspected.

CNIs are key components of immunosuppressive therapy and are not usually discontinued during acute rejection episodes. Instead, their levels and potential toxicity are closely monitored, and dosages may be adjusted. The decision to modify or withdraw these drugs is complex and depends on individual patient circumstances, including the severity of rejection and the overall immunosuppressive regimen.

Test 1 Questions

(1) Which of the following is true about the reabsorption of amino acids?

(A) Just like glucose, amino acids are also partially reabsorbed along with sodium.

(B) Amino acids are reabsorbed at the distal convoluted tubule through a passive transport mechanism.

(C) Amino acids are completely reabsorbed along with sodium from the proximal convoluted tubule through a secondary active transport mechanism.

(D) Amino acids are also completely reabsorbed along with potassium from the collecting duct under the effect of aldosterone.

(2) Which of the following is true about tubular secretion?

(A) All parts of the renal tubule secrete the same molecules and substances.

(B) Examples of substances secreted include amino acids and glucose.

(C) Substances secreted at the proximal convoluted tubules include water.

(D) Examples include penicillin, derivatives of amino acids, and acids such as 5-hydroxy indole acetic acid and para-aminohipuric acid.

(3) Where does sodium reabsorption primarily occur in the kidneys?

(A) Only in the proximal tubule.

(B) Only in the loop of Henle.

(C) In both the proximal tubule and the loop of Henle.

(D) In the distal tubules and collecting ducts.

(4) Which of the following is not true about water reabsorption?

(A) The distal convoluted tubule and the collecting duct are normally not permeable to water.

(B) Reabsorption of water at the distal convoluted tubule and the collecting duct depends on the activity of the anti-diuretic hormone.

(C) The proximal convoluted tubule becomes permeable to water only in the presence of the antidiuretic hormone.

(D) Water reabsorption in the proximal convoluted tubule follows the reabsorption of sodium.

(5) Which of the following can explain the presence of glucose in urine?

(A) Glomerular filtrate glucose concentration is above the renal threshold for glucose.

(B) The renal threshold for glucose is 180 g/L in arterial blood, so lower glucose concentrations are excreted in the urine.

(C) Glomerular filtrate glucose concentration is below the renal threshold for glucose.

(D) None of the above.

(6) Which of the following is true about urine formation?

(A) It ends with glomerular filtration, where blood from the afferent arteriole passes through glomerular capillaries and then filtered into the Bowman capsule.

(B) It is a complex process involving a series of interrelated events and processes, which include the production of erythropoietin, thrombopoietin, and vitamin D.

(C) Most substances desired by the body are secreted from filtrate whereas substances not desired by the body are reabsorbed into the tubule.

(D) It is a complex process involving a series of interrelated events, which include glomerular filtration, tubular reabsorption, and tubular secretion.

(7) Which is a substance that is reabsorbed from the glomerular filtrate?

(A) Plasma proteins.

(B) Glucose and amino acids.

(C) Albumin.

(D) Globulins.

(8) Which of the following is true about glomerular filtration?

(A) Glomerular filtration is the last step in the formation of urine.

(B) It occurs across the tubular cell, which is made up of cuboidal epithelium.

(C) The glomerular filtrate includes all of the components of plasma, including plasma proteins.

(D) Glomerular filtration occurs across the filtration membrane.

(9) Which of the following is true about the filtration membrane?

(A) The filtration membrane is made up of the afferent capillary membrane, efferent artery basement membrane, and the parietal layer of the Bowman capsule.

(B) The glomerular capillary membrane is made up of a layer of cuboidal brush-border cells attached to the basement membrane. It does not have fenestrations.

(C) The basement membrane is formed by the split between the endothelium of the glomerular capillaries and the epithelium of the Bowman's capsule.

(D) The filtration membrane is made up of the glomerular capillary membrane, the basement membrane, and the visceral layer of the Bowman capsule.

(10) Which of the following transport mechanisms does the reabsorption of molecules across the tubular cells occur?

(A) Active transport only.

(B) Passive transport only.

(C) Active and passive reabsorption.

(D) Transcellular and paracellular route.

(11) What is the key system that contributes to renal damage in diabetic kidney disease?

(A) Immune system.

(B) Endocrine system.

(C) Renin-angiotensin system (RAS).

(D) Respiratory system.

(12) What is the main therapeutic goal in the management of diabetic kidney disease and prevention of end-stage renal disease (ESRD)?

(A) Control blood glucose.

(B) Reduce protein intake.

(C) Increase sodium intake.

(D) Administer diuretics.

(13) A 60-year-old diabetic patient asks about the target HbA1c level to prevent kidney disease. What level should you recommend?

(A) 6.0%.

(B) 7.0%.

(C) 8.0%.

(D) 9.0%.

(14) Which class of drugs is considered the first-line therapy for management of hypertension in diabetic patients with kidney disease?

(A) Diuretics.

(B) Beta-blockers.

(C) Angiotensin-converting enzyme (ACE) inhibitors.

(D) Calcium channel blockers.

(15) How can statins prevent chronic kidney disease in a 58-year-old diabetic patient?

(A) Increase sodium retention.

(B) Reduce serum levels of AGEs.

(C) Enhance glomerular permeability.

(D) Promote endothelial dysfunction.

(16) Which of the following is a contraindication for the use of metformin in patients undergoing dialysis?

(A) Hyperkalemia.

(B) Renal impairment.

(C) Hypertension.

(D) Anemia.

(17) Which of the following signs is not considered atypical in a diabetic patient who presents with renal impairment?

(A) Rapid GFR decline.

(B) Massive proteinuria.

(C) Active urine sediment.

(D) Decreased serum creatinine levels.

(18) What factor contributes to high blood pressure in a patient with chronic kidney disease (CKD)?

(A) Decreased sodium intake.

(B) Reduced arterial stiffness.

(C) Impaired sodium reabsorption.

(D) Elevated sodium intake.

(19) Which system plays a critical role in regulating blood pressure and responding to changes in dietary sodium intake?

(A) Immune system.

(B) Endocrine system.

(C) Renin-angiotensin-aldosterone system (RAAS).

(D) Nervous system.

(20) In chronic kidney disease (CKD), what role does the sympathetic nervous system activity play?

(A) Decreases renin secretion.

(B) Reduces tubular sodium reabsorption.

(C) Promotes vascular dilation.

(D) Contributes to hypertension.

(21) What is the most common method for staging chronic kidney disease?

(A) Glomerular Filtration Rate (GFR).

(B) Blood pressure measurements.

(C) Urinary protein levels.

(D) Serum creatinine levels.

(22) According to the Kidney Disease Improving Global Outcomes (KDIGO) classification, which chronic kidney disease stage is an eGFR between 45-59 mL/min/1.73m^2?

(A) Stage 1.

(B) Stage 2.

(C) Stage 3a.

(D) Stage 3b.

(23) A patient with stage 3b chronic kidney disease will likely have which of the following eGFR values?

(A) 60-89 mL/min/1.73m^2.

(B) 30-44 mL/min/1.73m^2.

(C) 15-29 mL/min/1.73m^2.

(D) Less than 15 mL/min/1.73m^2.

(24) Stage 5 chronic kidney disease is also known as which of the following?

(A) End-Stage Renal Disease (ESRD).

(B) Mild CKD.

(C) Moderate CKD.

(D) Severe CKD.

(25) Which of the following is a marker of chronic kidney disease?

(A) Hypertension.

(B) Hematuria.

(C) Proteinuria.

(D) Anasarca.

(26) Which of the following indicates an increased risk of progressive renal dysfunction in a patient with stage 2 chronic kidney disease?

(A) Increased eGFR after diagnosis.

(B) Proteinuria.

(C) Hematuria of unknown origin.

(D) Advanced age at diagnosis.

(27) Which of the following is the foremost cause of mortality in patients with end-stage renal disease?

(A) Anemia.

(B) Hypertension.

(C) Uremia.

(D) Cardiovascular complications.

(28) End-stage renal disease is commonly defined as a glomerular filtration rate (GFR) of less than what?

(A) 15 $mL/min/1.73m^2$.

(B) 25 $mL/min/1.73m^2$.

(C) 35 $mL/min/1.73m^2$.

(D) 45 $mL/min/1.73m^2$.

(29) A patient with stage 4 chronic kidney disease may require the administration of exogenous erythropoietin to manage which of the following complications?

(A) Anemia.

(B) Thrombocytopenia.

(C) Pancytopenia.

(D) Bone marrow suppression.

(30) Which of the following statements is false?

(A) Chronic kidney disease is an independent cardiovascular risk factor.

(B) Most chronic kidney disease patients eventually progress to end-stage renal disease.

(C) eGFR usually detects chronic kidney disease before any change to serum creatinine.

(D) Urinalysis is required in patients with eGFR levels less than 90 $mL/min/1.73m^2$.

(31) Which of the following is not criteria commonly used to define AKI?

(A) RIFLE criteria.

(B) KDIGO criteria.

(C) AKIN criteria.

(D) Framingham criteria.

(32) Which of the following is a primary cause of prerenal AKI?

(A) Direct structural damage to renal tissues.

(B) Urinary tract obstruction.

(C) Reduced blood flow without structural impairment of the kidneys.

(D) Nephrotoxic medications.

(33) Which of the following is a characteristic feature of CKD?

(A) Sudden onset with an abrupt decline in renal function.

(B) Symptoms usually develop suddenly.

(C) Gradual onset over an extended period.

(D) Oliguria/Anuria is commonly seen in early stages.

(34) Which of the following is a common cause of CKD globally?

(A) Infections.

(B) Hypertension.

(C) Trauma.

(D) Genetic disorders.

(35) Which of the following is a key characteristic of AKI?

(A) Its reversible nature.

(B) The presence of bilateral, small echogenic kidneys on ultrasound imaging.

(C) A persistent abnormality in kidney structure for more than three months.

(D) A gradual decline in kidney function over time.

(36) What is a characteristic feature of CKD-associated anemia?

(A) Increased production of erythropoietin.

(B) Decreased production of erythropoietin.

(C) Normal red cell production.

(D) Elevated hemoglobin levels.

(37) Which category of AKI accounts for approximately sixty percent of cases?

(A) Prerenal AKI.

(B) Intrarenal AKI.

(C) Postrenal AKI.

(D) None of the above.

(38) What percentage of the global population is affected by CKD?

(A) Over fifty percent.

(B) Over thirty percent.

(C) Over twenty percent.

(D) Over ten percent.

(39) What is the primary cause of postrenal AKI?

(A) Direct structural damage to the renal tissue.

(B) Urinary tract obstruction.

(C) Reduced blood flow without structural impairment of the kidneys.

(D) Renal ischemia.

(40) What is the primary cause of intrarenal AKI related to tubular damage?

(A) Renal ischemia.

(B) Hemorrhage.

(C) Retroperitoneal fibrosis.

(D) Congestive cardiac failure.

(41) Which of the common complications of kidney disease presents with fatigue, poor tolerance to exercise, and decreased cognition and mental acuity?

(A) Anemia.

(B) Hypertension.

(C) Hypokalemia.

(D) Metabolic acidosis.

(42) You're the nurse on duty and receive laboratory results for Ms. Brown who is a known kidney disease patient. The suggestion is to give her phosphate binders. What could Ms. Brown be experiencing?

(A) Hypertension.

(B) Hyperkaliemia.

(C) Hypercalcemia.

(D) Hyperphosphatemia.

(43) A 54-year-old woman with kidney disease comes to the office because she has been feeling fatigue, itching, and a metallic taste in her mouth for the past two weeks. Respirations are 32/min. This patient's symptoms most likely show presence of which of the following conditions?

(A) Hypokalemia.

(B) Primary metabolic acidosis.

(C) Primary metabolic alkalosis.

(D) Primary respiratory acidosis.

(44) A patient with kidney disease who develops severe shortness of breath and fluid retention with hypertension that started in the early course of kidney disease is likely to have which of the following?

(A) Anemia.

(B) Heart failure.

(C) Metabolic acidosis.

(D) Hypertension.

(45) If a patient is undergoing dialysis, low levels of vitamin D can cause which of the following complications?

(A) Increased risk of infectious diseases.

(B) Secondary hyperparathyroidism.

(C) Hypotension during dialysis sessions.

(D) Excessive weight gain.

(46) Mr. Russel is a 62-year-old man with kidney disease. He has been experiencing high blood pressure that is difficult to control. What is associated with this condition in this patient?

(A) Cardiovascular disease.

(B) Increased risk of infection.

(C) Peripheral neuropathy.

(D) Metabolic acidosis.

(47) In patients undergoing dialysis, which factor is most commonly associated with the development of left ventricular hypertrophy (LVH)?

(A) Hypocalcemia.

(B) Hypertension.

(C) Hypernatremia.

(D) Hypokalemia.

(48) What risk factors predispose a patient with chronic kidney disease to cardiovascular disease as a complication?

(A) Low blood lipid profiles.

(B). Reduced inflammatory response.

(C) Increased oxidative stress and vascular damage.

(D) Increase in insulin.

(49) A kidney disease patient aged 62 complains of palpitations and a nurse finds her pulse to be irregular. Which type of heart complication is this?

(A) Low blood pressure.

(B) Hypoglycemia.

(C) Arrhythmia (atrial fibrillation).

(D) High HDL cholesterol.

(50) Vincent is a 49-year-old male with anemia and kidney disease. He was requested to go for echocardiography imaging because his heart appeared large on a chest x-ray. The results showed left ventricular hypertrophy (LVH). What condition might cause this?

(A) Anemia.

(B) Autoimmune disease.

(C) Metabolic acidosis.

(D) A bone disorder.

(51) What is the primary cause of anemia in patients with Chronic Kidney Disease who undergo dialysis?

(A) Reduced erythropoietin production by the kidneys.

(B) Excessive iron absorption in the gastrointestinal tract.

(C) Increased destruction of red blood cells in the spleen.

(D) Overproduction of hepcidin in the liver.

(52) A 43-year-old patient admitted to emergency with the diagnosis of AKI secondary to ATN begins to experience vomiting, uremic fetor, and bizarre behaviors. The attending nurse to the patient suspects the symptoms are due to uremic encephalopathy. Assessment of which of the following kidney functions will help her diagnose uremic encephalopathy?

(A) Secretory function.

(B) Excretory function.

(C) Regulatory function.

(D) Metabolic function.

(53) Which component of urine analysis measures parameters such as pH, glucose, albumin, and ketone?

(A) Gross assessment.

(B) Urine dipstick.

(C) Microscopy.

(D) Urine analysis has no role in determining pH, glucose, albumin, and ketone.

(54) Which one of the following conditions decreases BUN regardless of the GFR?

(A) Dehydration.

(B) High protein diet.

(C) Use of glucocorticoids.

(D) SIADH.

(55) Which one of the following imagining modalities is the gold standard for diagnosing nephrolithiasis?

(A) Ultrasound.

(B) Non-contrast CT scan.

(C) MRI.

(D) Contrast-enhanced CT scan.

(56) A patient admitted to your hospital after presenting with a complaint of flank mass of 7 months duration is ordered to have a contrast-enhanced abdominopelvic CT scan by the nephrologist. Which one of the following investigations is a prerequisite before performing the CT scan?

(A) Urine analysis.

(B) RFT.

(C) Echocardiography.

(D) Abdominopelvic ultrasound.

(57) Which one of the following conditions is not an indication to perform a kidney biopsy?

(A) Nephrotic syndrome in older children and adults.

(B) Acute nephritic syndrome.

(C) Unexplained acute kidney injury.

(D) Uremic encephalopathy.

(58) Which one of the following statements regarding kidney biopsy is not correct?

(A) It can result in life-threatening complications.

(B) Unexplained acute kidney injury is an indication to perform kidney biopsy.

(C) Patients require CBC and coagulation profile before the procedure to assess bleeding tendency.

(D) It can be performed by any health professional if an ultrasound is available.

(59) Which one of the following is not part of appropriate post-procedural care after a renal biopsy?

(A) Perform an MRI scan to rule out the presence of perinephric bleeding.

(B) Monitor vital signs serially immediately after the procedure.

(C) Keep the patient supine for 4 to 6 hours.

(D) Watch for flank pain and hematuria.

(60) Which of the following is a common sign of hemodialysis access dysfunction in patients?

(A) Decreased access site bleeding after dialysis.

(B) Increased blood flow through the access site.

(C) Prolonged bleeding from the access site after dialysis.

(D) Reduced sensation of warmth around the access site.

(61) End-stage renal disease is defined as:

(A) Glomerular filtration rate of less than 15mL/minute.

(B) Glomerular filtration rate of 60mL/minute.

(C) Temporary damage to the glomeruli.

(D) Marked reduction in urine production.

(62) Which of the following statements is true about hemodialysis?

(A) Hemodialysis is a cure for chronic renal failure and ESRD.

(B) A patient must receive in-center dialysis once a diagnosis of ESRD is made.

(C) Dialysis can affect the quality of life of the patient.

(D) A patient with ESRD on hemodialysis does not require a renal transplant.

(63) During hemodialysis, the following are filtered out from the body:

(A) Urine and other fluids.

(B) Blood, urine, and fluids.

(C) Water, urea, and creatinine.

(D) Poisonous substances.

(64) Hemodialysis works by simple:

(A) Absorption.

(B) Diffusion.

(C) Convection.

(D) Conduction.

(65) The following are types of modalities of hemodialysis except:

(A) In-center nocturnal hemodialysis.

(B) Conventional hemodialysis.

(C) Short daily hemodialysis.

(D) Peritoneal dialysis.

(66) The decision to administer a particular type of hemodialysis depends on all of the following except:

(A) The patient's history.

(B) The type of vascular access.

(C) The patient's sex.

(D) The patient's age.

(67) Which of the following is not true about conventional hemodialysis?

(A) Done six to seven times a week.

(B) Most common treatment worldwide.

(C) Sessions last up to three hours.

(D) Does not fully replace kidney function.

(68) Hemodiafiltration operates on the principle of:

(A) Diffusion.

(B) Diffusion and convection.

(C) Convection only.

(D) None of the above.

(69) The dialysate or dialysis fluid is made up of:

(A) Toxins.

(B) Blood and toxins.

(C) Water, sodium, and bicarbonate.

(D) Urine.

(70) One of the limitations of conventional hemodialysis is:

(A) Higher rates of hospitalizations in patients.

(B) Correction of fluid and electrolyte imbalance.

(C) Removal of body toxins.

(D) Can be done at home or in-center.

(71) Which of these is the primary objective of pre-dialysis assessment?

(A) Choose the best dialysis machine for the patient.

(B) Assess the patient's physiological state and health.

(C) Prepare the patient for palliative care.

(D) Prepare the patient for renal replacement therapy.

(72) What laboratory investigation analyzes renal function in pre-dialysis assessment?

(A) Serum bilirubin.

(B) Serum creatinine.

(C) Serum ferritin.

(D) Serum lipase.

(73) What lifestyle modification is vital for blood pressure management in pre-dialysis assessment?

(A) High-carbon diet.

(B) High-sodium diet.

(C) Low-sodium diet.

(D) Low-carbon diet.

(74) What is the target blood pressure for pre and post-dialysis patients?

(A) Greater than or equal to 150/90 mmHg.

(B) Less than or equal to 140/90 mmHg.

(C) Equal to 150/90 mmHg.

(D) Less than or equal to 170/90 mmHg.

(75) Dialysis preparation of diabetic patients does not involve:

(A) Nutritional and dietary support.

(B) Blood sugar check.

(C) Evaluation of cardiac function.

(D) Unlimited carbohydrate consumption.

(76) Which of the following statements regarding vascular access for hemodialysis is incorrect?

(A) It has two access points.

(B) A central venous catheter is preferred for emergency dialysis.

(C) Maturation failure after AVF creation occurs in around 80% of patients.

(D) AVG is more difficult to remove when compared to AVF.

(77) Which measures should not be taken to decrease access failure and its associated morbidity?

(A) Identify access at risk for thrombosis and failure.

(B) Maximize the use of AVG over AVF.

(C) Plan AVF formation as early as possible in CKD patients.

(D) Decrease the occurrence of access site infections and thrombosis.

(78) Mr. Wilson is a 62-year-old CKD patient attending your dialysis center. He needs long-term hemodialysis, and you explain AVF to him. When would you tell him to have the AVF done before the initiation of the hemodialysis?

(A) On the day of the HD.

(B) A day before the HD.

(C) A week before the HD.

(D) Two months before the HD.

(79) What is the gold standard investigation modality to decide the type and location of AVF?

(A) X-ray.

(B) Duplex ultrasound.

(C) CT angiogram.

(D) MRI.

(80) What is the most common complication associated with AVF?

(A) Maturation failure.

(B) Thrombosis.

(C) Aneurysm.

(D) Steal syndrome.

(81) Which one of the following vascular access options provides long-term and reliable access with minimal complications?

(A) AVF.

(B) AVG.

(C) Central venous catheter.

(D) All three have comparable longevity and complication rates.

(82) Laurel is a nurse at Mount Sinai's dialysis center. She explains the advantages of AVG over AVF to a patient. Which of the following statements regarding the advantages of AVG over AVF is correct?

(A) Less extensive surgery.

(B) Less risk of infection and thrombosis.

(C) Longer duration of use.

(D) Early use after creation.

(83) A nurse inserted a central catheter into the jugular vein of a patient requiring emergency hemodialysis to indicate uremic encephalopathy. What is the next appropriate thing to do?

(A) Proceed with the HD.

(B) Wait two hours before the initiation of HD.

(C) Perform a chest x-ray to ensure correct placement.

(D) Perform a chest CT scan to ensure correct placement.

(84) A nurse plans to insert a central venous catheter for a patient who requires an urgent HD. However, she has a high clinical suspicion that he might need permanent access soon. Which one of the following veins should the nurse avoid?

(A) Internal Jugular vein.

(B) Subclavian vein.

(C) Femoral vein.

(D) All three veins can be used with no future consequences.

(85) Which of the following statements regarding the advantages of central venous catheters is correct?

(A) They are difficult to insert.

(B) They are expensive when compared to AVF and AVG

(C) They can be used immediately.

(D) They are difficult to change.

(86) Which of the following best describes the purpose of the dialysate solution in hemodialysis?

(A) To clean the dialysis machine.

(B) To keep the patient hydrated.

(C) To remove waste and excess fluids from the blood.

(D) To provide nutrients to the patient.

(87) Which of the following is a method to obtain vascular access for hemodialysis?

(A) Through an intravenous line in the arm.

(B) Through a nasal cannula.

(C) Through a urinary catheter.

(D) Through a dialysis catheter in the abdomen.

(88) Which of the following is the function of hemodialysis's arteriovenous (AV) fistula or graft?

(A) It is used to measure blood pressure during dialysis.

(B) It connects an artery and a vein to provide access for blood flow.

(C) It filters waste products from the blood.

(D) It serves as a backup access site in case of emergency.

(89) Which of the following blood composition is not removed during a hemodialysis session?

(A) Urea.

(B) Creatinine.

(C) Red blood cells.

(D) Potassium.

(90) What is the purpose of the routine heparin administered during hemodialysis?

(A) To prevent clotting in the dialyzer and tubing.

(B) To stimulate red blood cell production.

(C) To ensure optimal clotting factors filtration.

(D) To provide pain relief to the patient.

(91) How is the blood flow rate through the dialyzer controlled during hemodialysis?

(A) Adjust the temperature of the dialysate.

(B) Increase the pressure in the arterial line.

(C) Adjust the dialyzer size.

(D) Adjust the blood pump rate.

(92) Which term describes the process of excess fluid removal from the body during hemodialysis?

(A) Ultrafiltration.

(B) Osmosis.

(C) Diffusion.

(D) Dialysis clearance.

(93) During hemodialysis, which type of solution is used in the hemodialysis machine to create a concentration gradient for removal of waste products from the blood?

(A) Saline solution.

(B) Bicarbonate solution.

(C) Dialysate solution.

(D) Antibiotic solution.

(94) Which of the following parameters is monitored closely during hemodialysis to ensure patient safety and well-being?

(A) Blood glucose levels.

(B) Blood pressure.

(C) Urine output levels.

(D) Temperature.

(95) Which factor is a direct determinant in establishing the duration of a hemodialysis session for a patient?

(A) The patient's dietary preferences.

(B) The level of physical activity of the patient.

(C) The patient's dry weight.

(D) The type of dialyzer used in the session.

(96) Blood is continuously moved from the patient's vascular access point to the dialyzer and back into the body. Which component of hemodialysis is responsible for this process?

(A) The blood pump.

(B) The blood pressure monitor.

(C) The dialyzer.

(D) The control panel.

(97) What is the main purpose of the dialyzer?

(A) It monitors the patient's blood pressure.

(B) It controls the composition of the dialysate.

(C) It filters waste products and excess fluids from the patient's blood.

(D) It regulates the patient's fluid intake.

(98) A fifty-seven-year-old male patient who is new to dialysis asks how the blood will move from him to the machine and back into his body. What is the appropriate response?

(A) Via a nasogastric tube.

(B) Via a urethral catheter.

(C) Via an arteriovenous fistula.

(D) Via an endotracheal tube.

(99) A patient is scheduled for a dialysis session to address fluid retention. Which component of the dialysis machine will be used for this purpose during hemodialysis?

(A) The control panel.

(B) The dialyzer.

(C) The blood pump.

(D) The ultrafiltration control.

(100) Mr. Jefferson has been experiencing low sodium levels. A safety alarm sounds during his dialysis treatment. What is this safety alarm likely detecting?

(A) The patient's high heart rate.

(B) The patient's low body temperature.

(C) Blood clotting in the dialyzer.

(D) The patient's low blood pressure.

(101) During dialysate preparation, high-quality purified water is used. What is the rationale behind this in hemodialysis?

(A) It prevents contamination of the dialysate.

(B) It adds electrolytes to the patient's blood.

(C) It regulates the patient's temperature.

(D) It helps maintain the patient's blood pressure.

(102) Which dialyzer should be used to remove larger molecules such as beta 2-microglobulin efficiently?

(A) A parallel plate dialyzer.

(B) A highly permeable dialyzer.

(C) A low-flux dialyzer.

(D) A high-flux dialyzer.

(103) A sixty-five-year-old woman yet to undergo dialysis has a respiratory rate of thirty-two breaths per minute and complains of fatigue and itchiness. As an experienced nurse, you recognize these as symptoms of metabolic acidosis. How will dialysis correct the acidosis?

(A) It will prevent blood clotting.

(B) It will remove metabolic waste products.

(C) It will maintain the patient's electrolyte balance.

(D) It will buffer the patient's blood acidity with bicarbonate.

(104) A patient would like to know what the term dialysis refers to. Which option best describes it?

(A) Hemodialysis.

(B) Chemo dialysis.

(C) Liver dialysis.

(D) Pancreatic dialysis.

(105) Dialyzers have membranes through which toxins move from the blood to the dialysate. These membranes are usually made from:

(A) Polyethylene.

(B) Chitin.

(C) Cellulose.

(D) Polyvinyl chloride.

(106) Which is the most common complication of hemodialysis?

(A) Cardiac arrest.

(B) Arrhythmias.

(C) Hypotension.

(D) Dialysis-induced amyloidosis.

(107) Which of the following proteins is deposited in tissues of patients with chronic hemodialysis?

(A) Albumin.

(B) Globulin.

(C) ß2-microglobulin.

(D) Amylin.

(108) Which of the following statements about infection transmission in hemodialysis is true?

(A) It occurs typically at the start or end of the hemodialysis.

(B) It occurs only at the start and end of hemodialysis.

(C) It occurs before hemodialysis.

(D) It occurs after dialysis.

(109) Which is not the following cause or source of infection in hemodialysis?

(A) Proper hand hygiene.

(B) Cross contamination of instruments.

(C) Mishandling of intravenous medications.

(D) Inadequate disinfection of dialysis equipment.

(110) Which is the most common bacterial cause of infection in hemodialysis?

(A) *Neisseria* spp.

(B) *Shigella* spp.

(C) *Cryptococcus* spp.

(D) *Staphylococcus* spp.

(111) Which of the following is matched appropriately to its corresponding class?

(A) Bacteria–Hepatitis B virus.

(B) Fungi–*E. Coli*.

(C) Parasite–*Toxoplasma gondii*.

(D) Virus–*Pseudomonas aeruginosa*.

(112) A 50-year-old man with end-stage kidney disease while on hemodialysis appeared unresponsive without cardio-respiratory activity. What is the next appropriate step?

(A) Rush and inform the caregivers.

(B) Watch and observe.

(C) Start CPR and defibrillation.

(D) Vigorously stimulate the patient.

(113) What is the cause of cardiac arrest in patients on hemodialysis?

(A) Fluid and electrolyte imbalances.

(B) Arrhythmias.

(C) Underlying cardiac disorder.

(D) All of the above.

(114) Which of the following is true about arrhythmias?

(A) It is always life-threatening.

(B) It is neither life-threatening nor benign.

(C) It can be benign or life-threatening.

(D) All of the above.

(115) Which of the following diseases does not have symptoms such as palpitations, tachycardia, and chest pain?

(A) Cardiac arrest.

(B) Arrhythmias.

(C) Myocardial infarction.

(D) Angina.

(116) A 60-year-old hemodialysis patient with chronic kidney disease presents with low serum albumin level. The patient weighs 75 kg. What is the recommended daily protein intake for this patient?

(A) 150 grams.

(B) 75 grams.

(C) 120 grams.

(D) 82 grams.

(117) A 45-year-old woman on hemodialysis has experienced muscle wasting and lethargy. What term best describes this condition?

(A) Chronic fatigue syndrome.

(B) Anorexia.

(C) Malnutrition.

(D) Protein-energy wasting.

(118) A 70-year-old man on hemodialysis has just been diagnosed with severe protein-energy wasting. Which healthcare professional should be responsible to develop a nutritional plan for this patient?

(A) Hemodialysis nurse.

(B) Nephrologist.

(C) Dietitian.

(D) Primary care physician.

(119) A 55-year-old woman on hemodialysis is looking to increase protein intake. What type of meat is ideal for this patient?

(A) Hot dogs.

(B) Canned chili.

(C) Eggs.

(D) Processed meats.

(120) A 62-year-old male with a history of end-stage renal disease on hemodialysis has experienced hypoalbuminemia. His nephrologist recommends oral supplements. What is the primary benefit of oral supplements?

(A) Reduce sodium intake.

(B) Improve serum albumin levels.

(C) Aid in weight gain.

(D) Replace the need for regular meals.

(121) A 50-year-old woman with a history of polycystic kidney disease is on hemodialysis. She recently reported digestive symptoms after her doctor prescribed oral supplements to fix her low albumin levels. What is an appropriate alternative for this patient?

(A) Parenteral nutrition.

(B) Intravenous fluids.

(C) Intramuscular injections.

(D) Intradialytic parenteral nutrition.

(122) A 68-year-old patient on hemodialysis reports difficulties in adherence to the nutritional plan suggested by his doctor. What key step can motivate this patient to stick to the recommended diet?

(A) Use of a harsh tone to scare the patient of the complications.

(B) Frequent diet changes.

(C) Close follow-up with a certified dietitian.

(D) Encourage cheat days.

(123) As a certified dialysis nurse, it is important to recognize the signs of depression in hemodialysis patients. Which of the following symptoms is most commonly associated with depression in these patients?

(A) Increased appetite.

(B) Insomnia or hypersomnia.

(C) Hypertension.

(D) Polyuria.

(124) A 50-year-old male on hemodialysis struggles with his diet and fluid restrictions. The patient started hemodialysis 3 weeks ago. His records show that he expressed a strong emotional reaction and shouted, "It cannot be me!" when his physician announced the diagnosis. What's the likely contributing factor to this issue?

(A) Financial issues.

(B) Poor family support.

(C) Denial.

(D) Strict religious beliefs.

(125) A 55-year-old woman in her first year of hemodialysis reports poor self-esteem due to weight fluctuations and scarring. How can this phenomenon be explained?

(A) Patients experience severe physical symptoms.

(B) Patients are more likely to discontinue treatment during the first year.

(C) Identity alterations occur due to body image changes and dependence.

(D) Patients are at a higher risk of depression and anxiety.

(126) Vancomycin is one of the most commonly used drugs in the medical management of dialysis patients. Which of the following best describes vancomycin's mechanism of action?

(A) It inhibits the protein synthesis.

(B) It inhibits the 30s ribosome.

(C) It decreases gene transcription.

(D) It inhibits bacterial cell wall synthesis.

(127) When caring for a patient on hemodialysis who is also taking angiotensin-converting enzyme (ACE) inhibitors, a nurse should be particularly vigilant for the development of:

(A) Hyperkalemia.

(B) Hypoglycemia.

(C) Hypertension.

(D) Hypercalcemia.

(128) Which of the following is not the action of heparin?

(A) Antiplatelet action.

(B) Lipemia clearing action.

(C) Anti-fibrotic action.

(D) Anticoagulant action.

(129) A 54-year-old male with a known case of chronic kidney disease presents for dialysis. A routine blood sugar test is done, and a diagnosis of diabetes is made. He has a previous diagnosis of hypertension and is on dietary therapy. He is advised for the medical management of hypertension. Which of the following best describes the medical management for this patient?

(A) Calcium channel blocker.

(B) Beta blocker.

(C) Angiotensin-converting enzyme inhibitor.

(D) Angiotensin II receptor antagonist.

(130) A 52-year-old male presented to the OPD with fatigue, muscle weakness, and body ache. A detailed investigation was done, and he was found to have secondary hyperparathyroidism, as he has had chronic kidney disease for the last two years. He was prescribed cinacalcet. Which of the following best describes the mechanism of action of this drug?

(A) Cinacalcet lowers the parathyroid hormone level by inhibiting the calcium-sensing receptor in the parathyroid.

(B) Cinacalcet lowers the parathyroid hormone level by activating the calcium-sensing receptor in the parathyroid.

(C) Cinacalcet lowers the parathyroid hormone level by inhibiting the parathyroid sensing receptor in the parathyroid.

(D) Cinacalcet lowers the parathyroid hormone level by activating the parathyroid sensing receptor in the parathyroid.

(131) Lipid abnormality is one of the common problems among dialysis patients with chronic kidney disease. Fibric acid analogs such as gemfibrozil are commonly used for its management. Which of the following best describes the mechanism of action of this drug?

(A) It inhibits peroxisome proliferator-activated receptor alpha (PPAR-alpha).

(B) It activates peroxisome proliferator-activated receptor alpha (PPAR-alpha).

(C) It inhibits peroxisome proliferator-activated receptor beta (PPAR-beta).

(D) It activates peroxisome proliferator-activated receptor beta (PPAR-beta).

(132) A 49-year-old male with a known case of chronic kidney disease presented to the OPD for routine dialysis. The standard heparinization procedure was adopted in this patient for heparin administration. Which of the following best describes the standard heparinization procedure?

(A) Administer a bolus of heparin before the patient is connected to the extracorporeal circuit.

(B) Continuous infusion of heparin during hemodialysis.

(C) Intermittent infusion of heparin during hemodialysis.

(D) Administer a bolus of heparin before the patient is connected to the extracorporeal circuit and continuous infusion of heparin during hemodialysis.

(133) A 52-year-old male with a known case of chronic kidney disease presented to the OPD for routine dialysis. On examination, his blood pressure was 160/90 mm Hg on the right hand in a sitting position. Which antihypertensive agent is best suited for this patient?

(A) Monotherapy with an angiotensin-converting enzyme inhibitor, an angiotensin II receptor antagonist, or a beta blocker.

(B) Dietary restriction only.

(C) A loop diuretic.

(D) A combination of the two or three drugs mentioned above.

(134) Which of the following is a critical action for a certified dialysis nurse to take when managing a patient who is experiencing an anaphylactoid reaction during hemodialysis?

(A) Immediately increase the rate of dialysis to clear potential allergens.

(B) Administer a bolus of high-glucose solution.

(C) Stop the dialysis treatment and administer epinephrine, if prescribed.

(D) Encourage the patient to relax and practice deep breathing exercises.

(135) A 52-year-old male presented to the OPD for routine dialysis and is a known case of chronic kidney disease. On examination, his blood pressure was 160/90 mm Hg on the right hand in a sitting position. He was prescribed a calcium channel blocker. Which of the following is the mechanism of action of this drug?

(A) It inhibits the receptor-operative channel.

(B) It inhibits the leak channel.

(C) It inhibits voltage-sensitive L-type channels.

(D) It inhibits the current sensitive L-type channel.

(136) A 46-year-old male patient on his first post-transplant day was found to have a blood pressure of 150/100 mmHg and a protein-to-creatinine ratio of 3. Which of the following antihypertensive drugs should be the first line?

(A) Amlodipine.

(B) Metoprolol succinate.

(C) Enalapril.

(D) Spironolactone.

(137) As a certified dialysis nurse, it is important to understand factors contributing to post-transplant hypertension. Which of the following medications is a known contributor to the development of hypertension after a kidney transplant?

(A) Antibiotics.

(B) Diuretics.

(C) Steroids.

(D) Antivirals.

(138) A 56-year-old female patient on her fourth post-transplant day complained of bilateral lower extremity swelling and a decreased urine amount over one day. On physical examination, she had a BP of 150/110 mmHg and a temperature of 100.2°F (axillary). The rest of her vital signs were in the normal range. She had periorbital edema and grade III bilateral pitting edema. Her creatinine was increased by 2 mg/dl from the baseline on laboratory investigations. What is the next best step in the management of this patient?

(A) Methylprednisolone.

(B) Cyclosporine.

(C) Kidney graft biopsy.

(D) Muromonab.

(139) In renal transplant patients who are allergic to cotrimoxazole, which medication is often used as a first-line alternative for urinary tract infection (UTI) prophylaxis?

(A) Amoxicillin.

(B) Doxycycline.

(C) Ciprofloxacin.

(D) Nitrofurantoin.

(140) The tuberculin skin test returned a positive result for a 45-year-old male patient in his sixth post-transplant week. This patient has a medical history, which includes receiving the BCG vaccination. What should be done regarding latent TB prophylaxis for this patient?

(A) Avoid prophylaxis because the positive skin test probably results from the BCG vaccine.

(B) Perform a chest x-ray initially to confirm latent TB.

(C) Use the QuantiFERON assay to confirm latent TB before giving prophylaxis.

(D) Prophylaxis should be given regardless of BCG vaccination status.

(141) Which of the following medications is appropriate during the initial maintenance phase of immunosuppressive therapy after transplantation for a patient with an acute graft rejection episode?

(A) Daclizumab and sirolimus.

(B) Mycophenolate mofetil, cyclosporine, and prednisolone.

(C) Mycophenolate mofetil and azathioprine.

(D) Mycophenolate mofetil and prednisolone.

(142) A 37-year-old female patient on her ninth post-transplant day was accidentally exposed to a nurse with a primary varicella infection two days ago. What is the best next step of management for this patient?

(A) Oral ganciclovir.

(B) Varicella immunoglobulin.

(C) Oral acyclovir.

(D) IV acyclovir.

(143) It is important to understand the clinical manifestations in renal transplant patients. Is gross hematuria a common finding in renal transplant patients?

(A) Yes, because the transplanted kidney is often prone to bleeding.

(B) No, because gross hematuria is not a typical feature in stable renal transplant patients.

(C) Yes, as it is a standard side effect of immunosuppressive therapy.

(D) No, unless there is a complication such as graft rejection or infection.

(144) A 46-year-old male patient, in his second post-transplant month with positive CMV serology, visited the clinic due to watery diarrhea persisting for two days. This was accompanied by sporadic low-grade fever, slight abdominal discomfort, and regurgitation of consumed substances. On physical examination, he is febrile and has dry buccal mucosa. The laboratory result was as follows:

Leucocyte count: 2000/µl, creatinine: 1 mg/dl.

What is the best next step in the management of this patient?

(A) DNA PCR.

(B) Enzyme immunoassay to detect anti-CMV antibodies.

(C) Colonic biopsy.

(D) IV ganciclovir.

(145) A post-transplant patient presents with a rash along dermatomes and a fever, which suggests that the patient has herpes zoster. Which of the following treatments is appropriate for this condition?

(A) Oral acyclovir.

(B) Intravenous iron supplementation.

(C) Topical hydrocortisone cream.

(D) Oral prednisone.

(146) A 40-year-old female patient who had a smooth postoperative period on her fourth post-transplant day started complaining of abdominal pain. When her chart was checked, the 24-hour urine output was 600 ml. On physical examination, there is a bulge over the wound site, and she has diffused abdominal tenderness. Ultrasound revealed fluid collection in the retroperitoneum. The fluid was aspirated and sent for analysis. It showed elevated creatinine, with LDH of 80 IU/ml and protein of 0.7 mg/dl. What is the most likely diagnosis for this patient?

(A) Primary spontaneous bacterial peritonitis.

(B) Postoperative urine leak.

(C) Secondary bacterial peritonitis.

(D) Graft pyelonephritis.

(147) When managing a postoperative patient with a high urine output (250 ml/hr), how should a nurse avoid fluid overload?

(A) Administer fluids at the same rate as the urine output.

(B) Administer slightly less fluid than the urine output.

(C) Administer significantly more fluid than the urine output.

(D) Avoid administering any fluids until urine output decreases.

(148) Which of the following methods should you use to measure the status of kidney transplant patients at risk of peri-operative heart failure?

(A) Continuous EKG monitoring.

(B) Jugular catheterization.

(C) Right heart catheterization.

(D) They do not need special monitoring.

(149) Which of the following is not true about managing patients with new-onset diabetes after transplantation (NODAT)?

(A) Aspirin should be prescribed for primary CVD prevention.

(B) The immunosuppressive treatment regimen should be modified to ameliorate diabetes.

(C) A HBA1C of ≤6% should be targeted for optimal treatment.

(D) Fasting blood sugar should be monitored weekly for one month for non-diabetic kidney transplant recipients.

(150) When counseling male kidney transplant recipients regarding fertility and medication safety, how should a nurse discuss the use of azathioprine?

(A) Advise against azathioprine due to the high risk of infertility.

(B) Inform that azathioprine is relatively safe in terms of fertility.

(C) Suggest azathioprine as a method to enhance fertility.

(D) Recommend azathioprine only for short-term use due to fertility concerns.

Test 1 Answers and Explanations

(1) (C) Amino acids are completely reabsorbed from the proximal convoluted tubule through a secondary active transport mechanism.

Just like glucose, amino acids are completely reabsorbed along with sodium from the proximal convoluted tubule through a secondary active transport mechanism.

(2) (D) Examples include penicillin, derivatives of amino acids, and acids such as 5-hydroxy indole acetic acid and para-aminohippuric acid.

Tubular secretion involves the transportation of molecules from blood into renal tubules. Examples include drugs such as penicillin, derivatives of amino acids, and acids such as 5-hydroxy indole acetic acid and para-aminohippuric acid. Different parts of the renal tubule secrete different molecules and substances. Molecules and substances secreted at the proximal convoluted tubules include potassium, ammonia, and hydrogen ions, whereas those secreted at distal convoluted tubules are potassium, minimal hydrogen ions, and urea at the loop of Henle.

(3) (C) In both the proximal tubule and the loop of Henle.

Sodium reabsorption in the kidneys is a process for maintaining electrolyte balance and blood pressure. A significant amount of sodium reabsorption occurs in the proximal tubule. Approximately 65-70% of the filtered sodium is reabsorbed in this part of the nephron. The reabsorption here is not under hormonal control and occurs alongside the reabsorption of other substances like glucose, amino acids, and bicarbonate. The loop of Henle uses a countercurrent multiplication mechanism to create a concentration gradient in the medulla of the kidney, which is crucial for water reabsorption in other parts of the nephron.

(4) (C) The proximal convoluted tubule becomes permeable to water only in the presence of the antidiuretic hormone.

Water reabsorption in the proximal convoluted tubule follows the reabsorption of sodium, as sodium creates a gradient that causes water osmosis. The distal convoluted tubule and the collecting duct are normally not permeable to water; however, they become permeable to water in the presence of the antidiuretic hormone. The reabsorption of water from these regions depends on the activity of the antidiuretic hormone, which stimulates the water channels known as aquaporins to increase water reabsorption.

(5) (A) Glomerular filtrate glucose concentration is above the renal threshold for glucose.

The renal threshold for glucose is 180 mg/dL in venous blood, so higher glucose concentrations are not reabsorbed but excreted in the urine.

(6) (D) It is a complex process involving a series of interrelated events, which include glomerular filtration, tubular reabsorption, and tubular secretion.

Urine formation starts with glomerular filtration, where blood from the afferent arteriole passes through glomerular capillaries, and then filtered into the Bowman capsule. Most substances desired by the body are reabsorbed from the filtrate, whereas substances not desired by the body are secreted into the tubule.

(7) (B) Glucose and amino acids.

Most substances desired by the body such as water, electrolytes, glucose, and amino acids are reabsorbed from the filtrate in the tubules. Substances not desired by the body are secreted into the tubule from peritubular blood vessels. Plasma proteins do not pass through the filtration membrane because of their size.

(8) (D) Glomerular filtration occurs across the filtration membrane.

Glomerular filtration is the first step in the formation of urine. It involves the filtration of blood across the filtration membrane, which is made up of glomerular capillary membrane, basement membrane, and the visceral layer of Bowman capsule. All of the plasma's components are filtered through except for the plasma proteins due to their huge molecular size, which is greater than the slit holes found in the endothelium of capillaries.

(9) (D) The filtration membrane is made up of the glomerular capillary membrane, the basement membrane, and the visceral layer of the Bowman capsule.

The glomerular capillary membrane is made up of a layer of endothelial cells attached to the basement membrane and has fenestrations with a diameter of about 0.1 μ. The basement membrane is formed by the fusion of the endothelium of glomerular capillaries and the epithelium of the Bowman's capsule.

(10) (C) Active and passive reabsorption.

Reabsorption across the tubular cells occurs by active reabsorption and passive reabsorption. In active reabsorption, molecules move against electrochemical or concentration gradient, which requires energy. In passive reabsorption, the molecules are transported along the concentration and electrochemical gradient. Reabsorption of molecules from the renal tubular lumen to the peritubular capillary occurs either through the transcellular route, where the molecules move through the cell, or the para-cellular route where molecules move through the intercellular space.

(11) (C) Renin-angiotensin system (RAS).

The key system that contributes to renal damage in diabetic kidney disease is the renin-angiotensin system (RAS). In diabetic kidney disease, the RAS is overactive, which causes hypertension and glomerular injury. Elevated renin and aldosterone levels precipitate increased sodium reabsorption and vasoconstriction of efferent arterioles, which damage the kidneys.

The immune system essentially deals with the body's defense against infections. However, it could be the culprit mechanism in autoimmune kidney disease. The endocrine system regulates hormones but does not play a role in kidney damage. The lungs are involved in respiration and gas exchange.

(12) (A) Control blood glucose.

The goal in the management of diabetic kidney disease is to control blood glucose levels. This helps prevent further kidney damage and the progression to ESRD.

Although protein intake may be part of the treatment plan, it is not the key focus for prevention of ESRD. Additionally, increased sodium intake is generally discouraged in diabetic kidney disease as it can exacerbate hypertension and kidney damage. The administration of diuretics is helpful for reduction of fluid overload that manifests as pulmonary edema or lower extremity swelling.

(13) (B) 7.0%.

The recommended target HbA1c level to prevent kidney disease progression is 7.0%. This level helps control blood sugar without risking hypoglycemia.

The first answer suggests a HbA1c level of 6.0%, which is ideal for healthy non-diabetic patients. The third and fourth options recommend looser control, which can further damage the kidneys and accelerate renal failure.

(14) (C) Angiotensin-converting enzyme (ACE) inhibitors.

The first-line therapy for the management of hypertension in diabetic patients with kidney disease is angiotensin-converting enzyme (ACE) inhibitors. ACE inhibitors slow down kidney disease progression in these patients.

Despite the usefulness of diuretics in edema, they are not the first-line choice. Beta-blockers are an alternative option but not the initial choice. Remember that beta-blockers are contraindicated in patients with asthma. Calcium channel blockers, however, are ideal for non-Caucasian hypertensive patients.

(15) (B) Reduce serum levels of AGEs.

Statins slow down the progression of chronic kidney disease in diabetic patients through reduction of the levels of advanced glycation end products (AGEs). These complex molecules have destructive properties that damage renal tissues.

(16) (B) Renal impairment.

Metformin is an oral antidiabetic medication commonly used in the treatment of type 2 diabetes. However, it has contraindications in certain conditions, one of which is significant renal impairment.

(17) (D) Decreased serum creatinine levels.

In a diabetic patient with renal impairment, decreased serum creatinine is not considered atypical. Serum creatinine levels typically rise due to reduced kidney function. The first, second, and third options all describe atypical signs of renal impairment in diabetic patients.

(18) (D) Elevated sodium intake.

Elevated sodium intake contributes to high blood pressure in patients with chronic kidney disease (CKD). Impaired sodium excretion causes elevated sodium levels and worsens blood hypertension.

Decreasing sodium intake is recommended in CKD management to alleviate hypertension. Reduced arterial stiffness is not a main contributor to high blood pressure in CKD. Impaired sodium reabsorption actually contributes to sodium retention and hypertension in CKD.

(19) (C) Renin-angiotensin-aldosterone system (RAAS).

The renin-angiotensin-aldosterone system (RAAS) plays a critical role in the regulation of blood pressure and responds to changes in dietary sodium intake.

(20) (D) Contributes to hypertension.

Upregulated sympathetic nervous system activity contributes to hypertension in chronic kidney disease (CKD). Increased renal sympathetic activity increases renin secretion, tubular sodium reabsorption, and vascular constriction, which raise blood pressure.

(21) (A) Glomerular Filtration Rate (GFR).

The glomerular filtration rate is a component of the renal excretory function and is widely accepted as the best overall index of kidney function. Most other kidney functions decline in parallel with eGFR in chronic kidney disease. Additionally, other parameters such as albumin-creatinine ratio (ACR) and albumin excretion rate over 24 hours can be used to stage chronic kidney disease.

(22) (C) Stage 3a.

The stages of CKD are classified according to the eGFR as follows:

- Stage 1: Kidney damage with normal or increased eGFR.
- Stage 2: Mild reduction in eGFR.
- Stage 3a: Moderate reduction in eGFR.
- Stage 3b: Moderate reduction in eGFR.
- Stage 4: Severe reduction in eGFR.
- Stage 5: Kidney failure.

(23) (B) 30-44 mL/min/1.73m^2.

The stages of CKD are classified according to the eGFR as follows:

- Stage 1: Kidney damage with normal or increased eGFR.

- Stage 2: Mild reduction in eGFR.
- Stage 3a: Moderate reduction in eGFR.
- Stage 3b: Moderate reduction in eGFR.
- Stage 4: Severe reduction in eGFR.
- Stage 5: Kidney failure.

(24) (A) End-stage Renal Disease (ESRD)

Stage 5 chronic kidney disease (also called end-stage renal disease, end-stage kidney disease, or kidney failure) occurs when the eGFR is less than 15 mL/min/1.73m^2. It is an indication for renal replacement therapy, which could be hemodialysis, peritoneal dialysis, or renal transplant.

(25) (C) Proteinuria.

A common marker of chronic kidney disease is proteinuria, which is generally first detectable as microalbuminuria. This is an albumin excretion of more than 30mg in 24 hours. Due to the difficulty of measuring 24-hour urine protein excretion, patients are often screened for proteinuria using a dipstick or a spot urine albumin-creatinine ratio. Other indicators of chronic kidney disease include abnormal urine sediment or abnormal imaging studies.

(26) (B) Proteinuria.

Factors that indicate an increased risk of advancing to more severe stages of kidney disease include the following.

- Proteinuria.
- Hematuria that originates from the kidneys.

- Decreased glomerular filtration rate with a loss of 5 mL/min/1.73m^2 or more within a year or 10 mL/min/1.73 m^2 or more over five years.
- Diagnosis at an early age.
- Family history of renal failure.
- Resistant hypertension.

(27) (D) Cardiovascular complications.

Cardiovascular complications are acknowledged as the primary cause of death in individuals with end-stage renal disease (ESRD) and account for over 50% of fatalities during the first year of dialysis. Research has demonstrated that even individuals with mild-to-moderate renal disease face an increased risk of cardiovascular events. The mortality rate for ESRD patients exceeds 20% annually. Therefore, cardiovascular complication prevention is paramount in managing patients with chronic kidney disease.

(28) (A) 15 mL/min/1.73m^2.

Stage 5 chronic kidney disease (end-stage renal disease, end-stage kidney disease, or kidney failure) occurs when the eGFR is less than 15 mL/min/1.73m^2. It is an indication for renal replacement therapy, which could be hemodialysis, peritoneal dialysis, or renal transplant.

(29) (A) Anemia.

The severity of anemia in chronic kidney disease is directly related to the extent of kidney function loss because the kidneys play a crucial role in erythropoiesis. People with norm normal kidney function respond to hypoxia with increased erythropoietin production, which consequently boosts red blood cell production. Patients with CKD have a primary deficiency in erythropoietin production by interstitial cells of the kidneys. Thus, they may require the administration of exogenous erythropoietin.

(30) (B) Most chronic kidney disease patients eventually progress to end-stage renal disease.

Only a small proportion of patients with chronic kidney disease eventually progress to end-stage renal disease. Proteinuria (detectable with urinalysis) is an important marker of chronic kidney disease. It is also an important prognostic indicator for outcome and therapy as chronic kidney disease with proteinuria is more likely to progress to end-stage. There is usually a reduction in eGFR before any change to serum creatinine.

(31) (D) Framingham criteria.

Several sets of criteria have been used in research studies to define AKI. They include RIFLE, KDIGO, and AKIN criteria. Each has unique benefits and limitations. KDIGO is the most recent and most commonly used tool. Framingham criteria are not used for defining AKI but for assessing the risk of coronary heart disease in various populations.

(32) (C) Reduced blood flow without structural impairment of the kidneys.

Maintenance of normal kidney function is highly dependent on adequate blood flow to the kidneys (referred to as renal perfusion). In prerenal AKI, there is a disruption in renal perfusion, which results in decreased blood supply to the kidneys. This impairs the kidneys' ability to filter waste products and effectively regulate fluid and electrolyte balances.

(33) (C) Gradual onset over an extended period.

Unlike AKI, which is characterized by a sudden and often reversible decline in kidney function, CKD is marked by a gradual and persistent deterioration of renal function over an extended period.

(34) (B) Hypertension.

Hypertension is one of the two most common noncommunicable causes of CKD globally (along with diabetes mellitus). It accounts for five to twenty percent of cases and contributes significantly to the growing burden of CKD.

(35) (A) Its reversible nature.

The reversible nature of AKI is a key characteristic that distinguishes it from CKD. With prompt and appropriate intervention, many AKI patients have the potential to recover and restore normal kidney function.

(36) (B) Decreased production of erythropoietin.

Anemia is a significant complication of CKD that occurs due to the impaired and decreased production of erythropoietin. This hormone is mainly produced in the kidneys, although it can also be produced in small amounts by the liver. Its primary role is to stimulate the bone marrow to produce red blood cells (erythropoiesis). In patients with CKD, the kidneys do not produce sufficient erythropoietin due to impaired renal function.

(37) (A) Prerenal AKI.

Prerenal AKI is the most common cause of AKI, It accounts for approximately sixty percent of cases.

(38) (D) Over ten percent.

CKD affects over ten percent of the global population.

(39) (B) Urinary tract obstruction.

Postrenal AKI occurs due to anatomical obstruction in the urinary system, which may occur at the pelvis, ureters, bladder, or urethra. This obstruction hinders the normal unidirectional flow of urine, which creates increased intraluminal pressure that has several detrimental effects on the kidneys. These include hydronephrosis, increased risk of infections (due to collection of stagnant urine), impaired renal blood flow, and risk of permanent kidney damage if the obstruction persists over an extended period.

(40) (A) Renal ischemia.

Tubular damage in intrarenal AKI is commonly caused by renal ischemia. Hemorrhage and congestive cardiac failure both cause volume depletion, which impairs renal blood flow and causes prerenal AKI. Retroperitoneal fibrosis is an extrarenal cause of urinary tract obstruction that causes postrenal AKI.

(41) (A) Anemia.

Anemia is a complication that presents with nonspecific symptoms including fatigue, poor tolerance to exercise, and even angina. In kidney disease, this usually results from erythropoietin deficiency.

(42) (D) Hyperphosphatemia.

High phosphate levels can be managed using phosphate binders to help maintain balance. If left unchecked, these elevated levels can cause bone and mineral disorders.

(43) (B) Primary metabolic acidosis.

The patient's history includes several risk factors for an acid-base abnormality. Chronic kidney disease, diabetes mellitus, and vomiting all lead to primary metabolic acidosis.

(44) B) Heart failure.

This condition arises as a complication of fluid retention and overload secondary to hypertension or anemia in kidney disease. It presents with symptoms such as shortness of breath, edema, etc.

(45) (B) Secondary hyperparathyroidism.

Vitamin D plays a crucial role in calcium and phosphate metabolism. In the context of patients undergoing dialysis, low levels of vitamin D are particularly concerning because they can contribute to the development of secondary hyperparathyroidism. This condition occurs when the parathyroid glands produce too much parathyroid hormone in response to low calcium levels, which is a common issue when vitamin D is deficient. Vitamin D is essential for calcium absorption; without it, calcium levels can fall and prompt increased PTH production to compensate for the shortfall. This overproduction of PTH can cause various complications, including bone demineralization and cardiovascular issues.

(46) (A) Cardiovascular disease.

This is secondary hypertension in a known kidney disease patient that increases the risk of other cardiovascular complications like heart failure and arrythmias.

(47) (B) Hypertension.

Left ventricular hypertrophy is a common cardiac complication for patients who undergo dialysis and is most commonly associated with hypertension. LVH refers to the thickening of the myocardium (muscle) of the left ventricle of the heart. When blood pressure is high, the left ventricle must work harder to pump blood against the higher pressure in the vessels. Over time, this increased workload can cause the muscle of the left ventricle to thicken and become less efficient, leading to LVH.

(48) (C) Increased oxidative stress and vascular damage.

Kidney disease is associated with an inflammatory state and increased oxidative stress. These are risk factors for the development of cardiovascular disease.

(49) (C) Arrhythmia (atrial fibrillation).

Arrhythmias in chronic kidney disease can result from electrolyte imbalance, hormonal effects like aldosterone fibrosis, as well as hypertensive effects.

(50) (A) Anemia.

Enlargement and thickening of the heart's left ventricle is a consequence of anemia due to its high output effects on the heart. Left ventricular hypertrophy is a cardiovascular complication in kidney disease that can be due to hypertension or anemia in this patient.

(51) (A) Reduced erythropoietin production by the kidneys.

Anemia is a common complication in patients with Chronic Kidney Disease, especially those undergoing dialysis. The cause of anemia in these patients is the reduced production of erythropoietin by the kidneys. Erythropoietin is a hormone that is critical for the production of red blood cells. In CKD, the kidneys' ability to produce adequate erythropoietin diminishes as the disease progresses, which causes a decrease in red blood cell production.

(52) (B) Excretory function.

Excretion of urea is one of the most important excretory functions of the kidneys. Failure to do so will result in complications such as uremic encephalopathy, uremic gastritis, and uremic pericarditis.

(53) (B) Urine dipstick.

The urine dipstick is the component of urine analysis that detects various parameters including pH, specific gravity, heme, protein (albumin), glucose, ketones, leukocyte esterase, nitrite, and urobilinogen.

(54) (D) SIADH.

BUN levels increase in cases of dehydration, catabolic state, high protein diet, and the use of certain drugs like glucocorticoids and tetracycline (TTC). BUN levels decrease in liver disease, malnutrition, old age, and SIADH, regardless of GFR.

(55) (B) Non-contrast CT scan.

Non-contrast CT scan is the gold standard investigation to diagnose nephrolithiasis and urolithiasis. Around 80 to 90 percent of renal stones are radiopaque. This limits the role of ultrasound in the diagnosis of nephrolithiasis.

(56) (B) RFT.

Evaluating a patient's renal function before administration of contrast agents is very important as they can be nephrotoxic and potentially worsen existing renal conditions.

(57) (D) Uremic encephalopathy.

Even though the presence of uremic encephalopathy requires dialysis, it is not an indication to perform a kidney biopsy per se. Indications to perform kidney biopsy include nephrotic syndrome in older children and adults, suspected systemic lupus erythematosus patients, acute nephritic syndrome, and unexplained acute kidney injury.

(58) (D) It can be performed by any health professional if an ultrasound is available.

Kidney biopsy should only be performed by trained professionals as its accuracy relies heavily on the technique used and the procedure carries a risk of life-threatening complications.

(59) (A) Perform an MRI scan to rule out the presence of perinephric bleeding.

Appropriate post-biopsy care after renal biopsy must keep the patient supine for 4-6 hours, monitor vital signs every 15 minutes for the first hour and every 30 minutes for the next four hours, and watch for flank pain and hematuria.

(60) (C) Prolonged bleeding from the access site after dialysis.

One of the key signs of hemodialysis access dysfunction is prolonged bleeding from the access site after dialysis. This can indicate issues such as clotting or stenosis (narrowing) in the access, which impairs its function and can cause inefficient dialysis treatment.

Efficient hemodialysis requires a well-functioning vascular access that allows for the rapid movement of blood into and out of the dialysis machine. If there are issues with the access site, like clotting or narrowing, it may not only affect the efficacy of the dialysis treatment but also increase the risk of complications.

(61) (A) Glomerular filtration rate of less than 15mL/minute.

Based on the KDIGO 2012 guidelines, chronic kidney disease (CKD) is classified into five stages based on the glomerular filtration rate (GFR):

- Stage one: Kidney damage, but the GFR is normal (more than 90mL/minute).
- Stage two: A mild decrease in the GFR (60-89mL/minute).
- Stage three: A moderate reduction in the GFR (45-59mL/minute).
- Stage three: A moderate decrease in GFR (30-44mL/minute).
- Stage four: A severe decrease in the GFR (15-29mL/minute).
- Stage five: ESRD with GFR (less than 15mL/min).

(62) (C) Dialysis can affect the quality of life of a patient.

Dialysis can significantly impact patients' lives. Its effects permeate various aspects, which include family dynamics, personal relationships, career progression, financial strain, and reproductive health. The other statements are false. Hemodialysis is only a treatment for ESRD while awaiting renal transplant. A renal transplant is the definitive cure for ESRD.

(63) (C) Water, urea, and creatinine.

During the hemodialysis process, the accumulated surplus water and toxins—specifically urea and creatinine—that the kidneys have failed to remove are filtered out from the blood. This procedure aids in detoxifying and purifying the blood, normally performed by functioning kidneys.

(64) (B) Diffusion.

Hemodialysis works by the simple principle of diffusion. Toxins from the blood are filtered into the dialysate through a semipermeable membrane. The blood serves as the high concentration, while the dialysis fluid serves as the low concentration.

(65) (D) Peritoneal dialysis.

Peritoneal dialysis is a unique type in which the peritoneum is leveraged as a semipermeable membrane. This enables an exchange of fluids and dissolved substances between the blood and a dialysis solution, which facilitates the removal of waste products from the body. This is unlike hemodialysis, where vascular access is required for the exchange.

(66) (C) The patient's sex.

The patient's sex does not affect the treatment modality. Age, body surface area, vascular access, and medical history are key factors. These considerations may affect your decision between in-center or home dialysis or conventional or short daily therapy.

(67) (A) Done six to seven times a week.

Conventional dialysis is done only three to four times a week. The other options are all true for conventional hemodialysis.

(68) (B) Diffusion and convection.

Hemodiafiltration operates on both diffusion and convection.

(69) (C) Water, sodium, and bicarbonate.

The dialysate is made up of pure water, sodium, and bicarbonate. It is used in the filtering of toxins out of the blood.

(70) (A) Higher rates of hospitalizations in patients.

Many studies have shown the high rate of complications associated with the conventional hemodialysis modality. Patients have been shown to have increased risks of cardiovascular complications, which may result in hospitalization.

(71) (B) Assess the patient's physiological state and health.

Pre-dialysis assessment involves the holistic analysis of the patient's physiologic health status. The purpose of patient assessment is to determine if the patient fits the criteria for dialysis. This process hinges on the evaluation of vital signs, patient weight, hydration levels, and vascular access. It also encompasses the analysis of laboratory results alongside these vital signs.

(72) (B) Serum creatinine.

A serum creatinine test is used to assess the kidney function of ultrafiltration. It also helps to monitor renal changes over time. Furthermore, it monitors kidney function in patients who undergo dialysis. The normal serum creatinine for adult males is 0.6-1.2 mg/dl. For adult females, it is 0.5-1.1 mg/dl.

(73) (C) Low sodium diet.

A low-sodium diet reduces the risk of certain diseases, such as hypertension. The consumption of excessive sodium triggers increased blood pressure. It also worsens edema and fluid overload. Reducing sodium intake helps to lower blood pressure or even prevent it. A low-sodium diet is both cardio and renal-protective. It has protective features against liver disease.

(74) (B) Less than or equal to 140/90 mmHg.

The recommended blood pressure target pre or post-dialysis is a value of less than or equal to 140/90 mmHg. Some works of literature suggest a pre-dialysis of <140/90 mmHg and a post-dialysis of <130/80 mmHg. Hypertension is present in the majority of patients with CKD. Therefore, it becomes essential to monitor and manage hypertension to mitigate the risk of heart disease.

(75) (D) Unlimited carbohydrate consumption.

A diet high in carbohydrates is unsuitable for individuals who are pre-diabetic or diabetic. Increased consumption of carbohydrates directly correlates with elevated blood sugar levels, making it a poor choice for those preparing for dialysis due to diabetes. Instead, dietary recommendations for diabetics emphasize the inclusion of fruits, vegetables, and whole grains like wheat, oats, and brown rice. Proteins, sourced from eggs, chicken, and fish, are also beneficial for those managing diabetes.

(76) (C) Maturation failure After AVF creation occurs in around 80% of patients.

Even though maturation failure is the most common complication associated with AVF, it only occurs in 20-60% of patients. Other complications include thrombosis, aneurysm formation, and steal syndrome.

(77) (B) Maximize the use of AVG over AVF.

Vascular access problems and failures are important causes of morbidity and hospital admissions in patients with CKD. One of the most important measures to decrease this is to maximize the use of AVF since it can provide reliable, long-standing access to dialysis with minimal complications.

(78) (D) Two months before the HD.

AVF must be planned at least one or two months before starting hemodialysis to ensure proper fistula maturation.

(79) (B) Duplex ultrasound.

The gold standard investigation to decide on the type and location of the fistula is a duplex ultrasound scan, which allows the assessment of the arterial and venous diameters.

(80) (A) Maturation failure.

The most common complication of AVF is maturation failure, which occurs in 20-60% of patients. Other complications include thrombosis, aneurysm formation, and steal syndrome.

(81) (A) AVF.

The main advantage of a mature, carefully cannulated, and functioning AVF is that it can provide reliable, long-standing access to dialysis with minimal complications. Patients will have high satisfaction and a good quality of life while being cost-effective.

(82) (D) Early use after creation.

Even though AVF is far superior in many aspects compared to AVG, the advantage AVG has over AVF is that it can be used soon after creation. Early cannulation grafts can be used within 24 hours of creation, while standard grafts can be used after 2-4 weeks after creation.

(83) (C) Perform a chest x-ray to ensure correct placement.

A chest x-ray should be performed after insertion to confirm correct positioning before use for cuffed tunneled percutaneous catheters and vascular catheters placed in the internal jugular and subclavian veins.

(84) (B) Subclavian vein.

The possibility of subclavian stenosis, which could jeopardize future fistulas, should prevent any patients needing permanent access from undergoing the subclavian approach.

(85) (C) They can be used immediately.

The advantages of a central venous catheter include ease of insertion, low cost, ease of change, and immediate usability. The disadvantages include infection, venous stenosis or thrombosis, local complications, short life, and easy dislodgment.

(86) (C) To remove waste and excess fluids from the blood.

The main function of the dialyzer in hemodialysis is to eliminate waste products and excess fluids from the bloodstream. It acts as the artificial kidney and allows for the exchange of toxic substances between the patient's blood and the dialysate solution.

(87) (D) Through a dialysis catheter in the abdomen.

Before the commencement of hemodialysis, a vascular access point must be established. This can be done through arteriovenous fistula creation, an arteriovenous graft, or a catheter. Intravenous line via cannulation in the arm is not routinely used for dialysis.

(88) (B) It connects an artery and a vein to provide access to blood flow.

The arteriovenous (AV) fistula or graft function in hemodialysis provides a stable and efficient access point for the removal and return of blood during dialysis. These access sites are surgically created connections between an artery and a vein, mainly in the patient's arm. The AV fistula or graft allows for a higher blood flow rate. This makes it easier to circulate the blood through the dialysis machine and effectively remove waste products and excess fluids.

(89) (C) Red blood cells.

During hemolysis, waste products, excess fluids, and toxic substances are removed from the blood while the loss of essential components, such as proteins and red blood cells is minimized. As the patient's blood and dialysate flow through the dialyzer counter-currently, waste products, toxins, and excess fluids pass through the semi-membrane into the dialysate. At the same time, essential substances like erythrocytes and proteins remain in the blood.

(90) (A) To prevent clotting in the dialyzer and tubing.

The routine heparin administration during hemodialysis aims to prevent clotting in the dialyzer and the tubing that is part of the dialysis circuit. During hemodialysis, when the patient's blood is exposed to the dialyzer and tubing, there is a risk of clot formation due to contact with the foreign surfaces of the machine. Clotting can impede blood flow and reduce the effectiveness of the dialysis. The administration of heparin helps to maintain the blood's ability to flow smoothly through the dialyzer and tubing, prevents clot formation, and ensures efficient removal of waste products and excess fluids.

(91) (D) Adjust the blood pump rate.

The blood flow rate through the dialyzer during hemodialysis is controlled by adjustment of the blood pump rate. The blood pump is a component of the hemodialysis machine that draws blood from the patient's vascular access (an AV fistula or graft) and pushes it through the dialyzer, where waste products and excess fluids are eliminated from the blood before being returned to the body. Through regulation of the speed of the blood pump, healthcare providers can control the rate at which the patient's blood flows through the dialyzer, which allows for effective filtration and treatment.

(92) (A) Ultrafiltration.

Ultrafiltration is the term used for the process of excess fluid removal from the body during hemodialysis. It helps to maintain the patient's fluid balance and manage generalized edema, which is a common feature of chronic kidney disease.

(93) (C) Dialysate solution.

A "dialysate solution" is used in the hemodialysis machine to create a concentration gradient to remove waste products from the blood. The constituents of the dialysate solution can be adjusted based on the patient's individual needs and the goals of the treatment.

(94) (B) Blood pressure.

Blood pressure is monitored closely during hemodialysis to ensure patient safety and well-being. Maintenance of stable blood pressure is vital during the dialysis procedure because blood pressure fluctuations can adversely affect the patient's health. During hemodialysis, patients may experience fluid and electrolyte balance changes, which can impact blood pressure. Monitoring blood pressure allows healthcare providers to make real-time adjustments to the dialysis machine to help stabilize blood pressure and prevent complications like hypotension or hypertension.

(95) (C) The patient's dry weight.

The duration of a hemodialysis session is directly determined by the patient's dry weight, which is the weight of the patient after all excess fluid has been removed. Dry weight is a critical factor in hemodialysis, as it helps guide the amount of fluid that needs to be removed during the session. The goal of hemodialysis is to remove enough fluid to reach this dry weight without causing hypotension or other complications.

(96) (A) The blood pump.

The blood pump is responsible for circulating the patient's blood during hemodialysis. This is achieved through peristatic action aided by two low-voltage rollers which maintain a controlled flow rate.

(97) (C) It filters waste products and excess fluids from the patient's blood.

A dialyzer is also known as an artificial kidney. The dialysate and blood flow in opposite directions while waste flows from the blood into the dialysate.

(98) (C) Via an arteriovenous fistula.

An arteriovenous fistula is a type of access that is created for dialysis patients. An artery is surgically connected to a vein, which allows for efficient needle insertion for blood to be drawn out and returned during dialysis treatments.

(99) (D) The ultrafiltration control.

The ultrafiltration control component manages the removal of excess fluid from the body through the use of hydrostatic pressure across a semipermeable membrane of the dialyzer.

(100) (D) The patient's low blood pressure.

Patients with low sodium levels are prone to hypotension during dialysis. Blood pressure changes trigger safety alarms, as do the presence of air in blood tubes and other critical variable changes.

(101) (A) It prevents contamination of the dialysate.

To ensure purity and prevent contamination, water for hemodialysis undergoes filtration, softening, deionization, and reverse osmosis to remove microbiologic contaminants and dissolved ions. This prevents dialysis-associated infections and other problems.

(102) (D) A high-flux dialyzer.

High-flux dialyzers have high hydraulic permeability. They clear beta 2-microglobulin at a rate of ≥15 mL/min. Their large pores clear large molecules efficiently.

(103) (D) It will buffer the patient's blood acidity with bicarbonate.

Bicarbonate in the dialysate regulates pH by reacting with excess hydrogen ions in the blood, which forms carbonic acid that is converted to carbon dioxide and water. These end products are easily removed.

(104) (A) Hemodialysis.

The term dialysis means the filtering and removal of metabolic wastes from the blood. It commonly refers to the function of the kidneys. Thus, one would describe it as hemodialysis. Another type of dialysis that removes waste through the peritoneal lining is called peritoneal dialysis.

(105) (C) Cellulose.

Cellulose is biocompatible and readily available. It is commonly used in dialyzers because it is inexpensive and easily strengthened. Its pore size allows the efficient filtration of wastes.

(106) (C) Hypotension.

This is the most common acute complication of hemodialysis, with an incidence of 15–30%.

(107) (C) ß2-microglobulin.

Dialysis-related amyloidosis is characterized by the deposition of amyloid ß2-microglobulin in different body tissues.

(108) (A) It occurs typically at the start or end of the hemodialysis.

Infection transmission in hemodialysis can occur at any time, but it typically occurs during the start and/or at the end of the hemodialysis session.

(109) (A) Proper hand hygiene.

Sources of infections in hemodialysis include improper hand hygiene, cross-contamination of instruments, mishandling of intravenous medications, inadequate disinfection of dialysis equipment, poor or nonadherence to infection prevention and control standard practices, and suppressed immunity.

(110) (D) *Staphylococcus* spp.

The common bacterial pathogens in hemodialysis are *Staphylococcus aureus,* coagulase-negative staphylococci, *Pseudomonas aeruginosa, Escherichia coli, Klebsiella,* and *Enterobacter.*

(111) (C) Parasite–*Toxoplasma gondii.*

A common parasitic pathogen implicated in hemodialysis infection is the *Plasmodia* species called *Toxoplasma gondii.*

(112) (C) Start CPR and defibrillation.

The appropriate immediate step to take after a cardiac arrest is cardiopulmonary resuscitation (CPR) and defibrillation.

(113) (D) All of the above.

Cardiac arrest in patients on hemodialysis is caused by fluid and electrolyte imbalances, arrhythmias, dialysis disequilibrium syndrome, and underlying cardiac disorders.

(114) (C) It can be benign or life-threatening.

Arrhythmias in hemodialysis can be relatively harmless or life-threatening.

(115) (A) Cardiac arrest.

Cardiac arrest is a sudden cessation of cardiac activity, and so there will not be arrhythmias, myocardial infarction, or angina.

(116) (D) 82 grams.

In the context of hemodialysis, protein intake is vital for patients. The recommended daily protein intake according to recent guidelines is 1.1 grams per kilogram of ideal body weight (IBW) per day. This is important to maintain muscle mass and overall health in hemodialysis patients. The math for this patient indicates 82.5 grams per day.

(117) (D) Protein-energy wasting.

Protein-energy wasting is a condition characterized by muscle atrophy and low energy levels, which is frequently seen in hemodialysis patients. It is caused by an inadequate supply of calories and protein to meet the body's needs.

(118) (C) Dietitian.

Creating a tailored nutritional plan for hemodialysis patients is a complex task that requires the expertise of a certified dietitian. Dietitians have the specialized knowledge to design dietary plans that meet the specific needs of patients with chronic kidney disease on hemodialysis. Although a primary care physician and nephrologist may aid in specific nutritional deficiencies when they become symptomatic, a comprehensive dietary plan requires a certified dietitian.

(119) (C) Eggs.

The best protein source for hemodialysis patients is rich in amino acids and low in sodium/phosphorus. This helps them increase their protein intake and manage their phosphorus intake, which is essential for kidney health. The first and second options are not recommended due to their high content of phosphorus. Processed meats also tend to be rich in sodium and phosphorus.

(120) (B) Improve serum albumin levels.

Oral nutritional supplements are beneficial for hemodialysis patients because they can improve serum albumin levels without the risk of adverse effects on electrolyte balance. These supplements provide essential nutrients and can help address protein deficiencies, which are common in this patient population. The reduction in sodium intake may be a desirable effect of oral supplementation.

(121) (D) Intradialytic parenteral nutrition.

For patients who have tolerability issues with oral nutritional supplements, the use of intradialytic parenteral nutrition (IDPN) is recommended. This type of supplementation is preferred for these patients and can help address their nutritional needs, especially when oral supplements are not well-tolerated. Parenteral nutrition and IV fluids are reserved for patients with severe malnutrition.

(122) (C) Close follow-up with a certified dietitian.

The key to promote adherence to nutritional guidelines for hemodialysis patients is close follow-up with a certified dietitian. Dietitians can provide ongoing support, guidance, and adjustments to the dietary plan to ensure that patients adhere to their nutritional requirements. This collaborative approach is vital for the overall well-being of hemodialysis patients. The first option suggests using an unpleasant tone to scare the patient. Although this may work for some patients, it can be problematic. Healthcare providers should also remember that they're not supposed to cause physical or psychological harm to the patient regardless of the circumstances. The final option for frequent cheat days can expose the patient to hypernatremia or hyperphosphatemia. These electrolyte imbalances can have dire consequences.

(123) (B) Insomnia or hypersomnia.

Depression is a common comorbidity in patients undergoing hemodialysis and can significantly impact their quality of life and treatment adherence. One of the key symptoms of depression in this patient population is a disturbance in sleep patterns, which can manifest as either insomnia or hypersomnia (excessive sleeping).

(124) (C) Denial.

Patients who recently started hemodialysis are at the greatest risk of denial. After being free for decades, it is extremely challenging to accept the diagnosis of ESRD and start hemodialysis with all its restrictions. Financial issues and poor family support could also be contributing factors. However, this patient is most likely dealing with denial. Refusing the treatment because of religious beliefs is found in a subset of patients.

(125) (C) Identity alterations occur due to body image changes and dependence.

The first year of hemodialysis is critical because patients may undergo identity alterations due to changes in body image and increased dependence. Although depression and anxiety can occur during the first year, they are more likely to present with other symptoms, such as anhedonia (i.e., loss of interest), insomnia, constant fear, and somatization of symptoms (e.g., tachycardia).

(126) (D) It inhibits bacterial cell wall synthesis.

Vancomycin and gentamicin are the most commonly used drugs in the medical management of dialysis patients. Gentamicin is derived from Micromonospora purpura. Vancomycin inhibits cell wall synthesis.

(127) (A) Hyperkalemia.

ACE inhibitors are medications commonly used in patients with chronic kidney disease for the management of hypertension and heart failure. However, one of the side effects of ACE inhibitors is the increased risk of hyperkalemia, which is an elevated level of potassium in the blood. This risk is particularly pronounced in patients with reduced kidney function, as the kidneys are less able to excrete potassium. Hemodialysis patients already have a compromised ability to regulate potassium due to their kidney disease, which makes the risk of hyperkalemia higher when they are on ACE inhibitors.

(128) (C) Anti-fibrotic action.

Heparin does not have anti-fibrotic action. Heparin is one of the most commonly used anticoagulants in dialysis patients and is a nonuniform mixture of mucopolysaccharides. The molecular weight of heparin is between 10,000 and 20,000 Da, and it contains polymers of D-glucosamine-L-iduronic acid and D-glucosamine-D-glucoronic acid. It has anticoagulant, antiplatelet, and lipemia-clearing properties.

(129) (C) Angiotensin-converting enzyme inhibitor.

Angiotensin-converting enzyme inhibitors (ACE inhibitors) are one of the most commonly used drugs to control hypertension in dialysis patients with end-stage renal disease. They are usually preferred if the patient also has left ventricular heart failure or endocrine manifestations like diabetes. It should be noted that anaphylactic reactions can occur in hemodialysis patients due to reactions with the AN69 membrane. This rare anaphylactoid reaction is unpredictable, and the group of antihypertensive drugs should be changed immediately if such reactions occur.

(130) (B) Cinacalcet lowers the parathyroid hormone level by activating the calcium-sensing receptor in the parathyroid.

Cinacalcet is one of the most commonly used drugs to manage secondary hyperparathyroidism in cases of dialysis. Cinacalcet decreases the level of parathyroid hormone. This action of cinacalcet is due to the activation of calcium-sensing receptors, which are normally in the parathyroid gland.

(131) (B) It activates peroxisome proliferator-activated receptor alpha (PPAR-alpha).

Fibric acid analogs like gemfibrozil are a commonly used drug to manage lipid abnormality in a patient undergoing dialysis. Gemfibrozil can lower the triglyceride level by activating peroxisome proliferator-activated receptor alpha. In the final run, it corrects the lipid abnormality in dialysis patients. However, in suspected or diagnosed cases of rhabdomyolysis, fabric acid should not be used in combination with statins.

(132) (D) Administer a bolus of heparin before the patient is connected to the extracorporeal circuit and continuous infusion of heparin during hemodialysis.

Guidelines have been created to ease the dose calculation and achieve the best coagulation profile in a dialysis patient. Initially, the patient should be given around 2,000-5,000 International Units of heparin. This dose can be given by opening a venous line or through other access lines. After administering the initial dose, it is important to wait two to three minutes so that the initial bolus mixes with the circulation uniformly. This is followed by continuous infusion of heparin at 500-1,000 International Units per hour. This maintenance dose can be given by opening an arterial line. During each of these processes, PTT is measured and monitored carefully.

(133) (A) Monotherapy with an angiotensin-converting enzyme inhibitor, an angiotensin II receptor antagonist, or a beta blocker.

The dosing and frequency of the antihypertensive drug depend on several factors, which include a patient's status and weight. A stepwise protocol has been developed for the systematic use of antihypertensive medications in these patients and includes the following steps:

Step 1: The patient is treated with monotherapy, such as AT1-angiotensin II receptor antagonists, angiotensin-converting enzyme inhibitors, or beta blockers.

Step 2: A loop diuretic is added if urinary output in this patient is high, i.e., more than 600 ml. Furosemide is the most commonly used drug among the loop diuretics.

Step 3: If the blood pressure is not controlled or maintained within the targeted limit by the agents mentioned above, then a two or three-drug combination can be added. A calcium channel blocker can be added in this step.

Step 4: A bilateral nephrectomy is only indicated if all the mentioned drugs and therapy fail to control the hypertension.

(134) (C) Stop the dialysis treatment and administer epinephrine, if prescribed.

An anaphylactoid reaction is a serious allergic reaction that can occur during hemodialysis, particularly in response to the dialyzer membrane or other components of the dialysis circuit. The initial and most critical action in managing such a reaction is to immediately stop the dialysis treatment to prevent further exposure to the allergen. Following this, the administration of epinephrine may be necessary, depending on the severity of the reaction. Epinephrine is a life-saving medication that can rapidly counteract the severe effects of anaphylaxis.

(135) (C) It inhibits voltage-sensitive L-type channels.

Calcium channel blockers do not affect leak or receptor-operated channels. They only block voltage-sensitive channels. These channels are present in smooth muscle cells. This group of agents has maximum efficacy in patients with coronary heart disease. An important precaution for the use of this drug is that it should not be used concurrently with beta blockers.

(136) (C) Enalapril.

ACE inhibitors and angiotensin receptor blockers (ARB) are the first-line drugs for patients with concomitant hypertension and proteinuria.

(137) (C) Steroids.

Steroids such as prednisone are used after a transplant to prevent organ rejection. However, one of the known side effects of steroid use is the development of hypertension. Steroids can increase blood pressure by causing fluid retention and affecting the balance of electrolytes, including sodium. Also, they can impact the responsiveness of blood vessels to vasoconstrictors, which further contributes to increased blood pressure.

(138) (C) Kidney graft biopsy.

The patient has fever, edema, hypertension, and rising serum creatinine, which are manifestations of acute graft rejection. The next appropriate step in managing this patient is a renal biopsy. Therapy is subsequently started after that. The drug of choice is methylprednisolone.

(139) (B) Doxycycline.

Cotrimoxazole (trimethoprim/sulfamethoxazole) is used for UTI prophylaxis in renal transplant patients because it prevents urinary tract infections, which are common complications after a transplant. However, in patients who have an allergy to cotrimoxazole, doxycycline is often used as a first-line alternative. Doxycycline is a tetracycline antibiotic that prevents infections due to its broad-spectrum antibacterial activity. Its use as an alternative to cotrimoxazole comes from its efficacy in preventing UTIs and its generally well-tolerated profile in patients who cannot take cotrimoxazole.

(140) (D) Prophylaxis should be given regardless of BCG vaccination status.

If a transplant patient has a positive tuberculin skin test or a positive result on an interferon-gamma assay, treatment for latent TB should be started regardless of BCG vaccine status since the effect of the BCG vaccine is unlikely to persist after ten years.

(141) (B) Mycophenolate mofetil, cyclosporine, and prednisolone.

A combination of an antiproliferative agent and a calcineurin inhibitor is given during the initial maintenance phase of immunosuppressive therapy. However, a steroid should also be added for a patient with an acute rejection episode. Daclizumab is an interferon-2 receptor antagonist, and it is used during the inductive phase.

(142) (B) Varicella immunoglobulin.

The KIDGO practice guideline recommends varicella or IV immunoglobulin as first-line prophylaxis for transplant patients exposed to primary varicella infection within four days of exposure.

(143) (B) No, because gross hematuria is not a typical feature in stable renal transplant patients.

Gross hematuria, which is visible blood in the urine, is not a common clinical manifestation in renal transplant patients who are stable. It may indicate other underlying issues such as urinary tract infections, graft rejection, or other complications related to the transplant.

(144) (A) DNA PCR.

The leucopenia and the signs and symptoms suggest an active CMV infection. He also has evidence of a previous infection. You can diagnose an active infection and viral load using DNA PCR. Serologic tests cannot differentiate between an acute infection and a previous one. Hence, they are useless in this case. Since other pathogens could present with similar manifestations, treatment should be started after the infection is confirmed.

(145) (A) Oral acyclovir.

Herpes zoster is known as shingles. It is a viral infection that is caused by the reactivation of the varicella-zoster virus. It is characterized by a painful rash that usually appears along dermatomes. In post-transplant patients, who are often on immunosuppressive therapy, there is an increased risk of viral infections such as herpes zoster. Oral acyclovir is an antiviral medication that helps to treat herpes zoster. It inhibits viral DNA synthesis and reduces the severity of the infection.

(146) (B) Postoperative urine leak.

This patient has a decreased urine amount with signs of peritonitis. The fact that there is fluid collection in the retroperitoneum with a high creatinine content is highly suggestive of a postoperative urine leak. The absence of ascitic fluid prior to presentation and the high creatinine and low LDH and protein content of the fluid are against peritonitis in this patient.

(147) (B) Administer slightly less fluid than the urine output.

In a postoperative patient who is experiencing a high urine output, such as 250 ml/hr, careful fluid management is necessary to avoid both dehydration and fluid overload. The goal is to replace lost fluids while maintaining a proper fluid balance. Administering fluids at a rate slightly less than the urine output (in this case, less than 250 ml/hr) helps in achieving this balance. This approach ensures that the patient is adequately hydrated without the risk of fluid overload, which can cause complications such as pulmonary edema or heart failure.

(148) (C) Right heart catheterization.

An intraoperative swan-ganz catheter should be placed in the right atrium to monitor the status of patients with cardiomyopathy or low (EF <40%) ejection fraction since they are at a high risk of peri-operative heart failure.

(149) (C) A HBA1C of ≤6% should be targeted for optimal treatment.

The optimal HBA1C target for patients with NODAT is 7 to 7.5%. A target HBA1C ≤6% would predispose the patient to hypoglycemia and thus should be avoided.

(150) (B) Inform that azathioprine is relatively safe in terms of fertility.

Azathioprine is an immunosuppressive medication that is used in kidney transplant recipients to prevent organ rejection. Research and clinical experience suggest that azathioprine does not significantly affect male fertility. This information is important for male patients who are concerned about their reproductive health after a transplant.

Test 2 Questions

(1) Which of the following is true about the reabsorption of bicarbonate?

(A) It is actively reabsorbed in the form of carbonic acid from the proximal convoluted tubule.

(B) It usually exists as carbonic acid in the renal filtrate.

(C) Sodium bicarbonate dissociates into water and bicarbonate, where the bicarbonate forms carbonic acid after combining with water.

(D) Sodium bicarbonate dissociates into sodium and bicarbonate, where the bicarbonate forms carbonic acid after combining with hydrogen.

(2) Which of the following is/are the functions of the kidney?

(A) It inhibits hormones such as erythropoietin, thrombopoietin, and renin.

(B) It excretes unwanted waste products such as glucose and amino acids.

(C) It produces vitamin K, which helps absorb calcium from the intestines.

(D) It excretes unwanted waste products such as urea, uric acid, creatinine, and bilirubin, as well as other substances such as drugs and toxins.

(3) Which of the following metabolism products is correctly matched?

(A) Urea generated from the degradation of hemoglobin.

(B) Creatinine generated from amino acid metabolism.

(C) Bilirubin generated from the metabolism of muscle tissue.

(D) Creatinine from muscle tissue.

(4) Which of the following is not true about the synthesis of vitamin D?

(A) Vitamin D3 is an active and important form of vitamin D.

(B) Vitamin D is synthesized in the skin from 7-dehydrocholesterol.

(C) The 7-dehydrocholesterol is converted by ultraviolet rays into 25-hydroxycholecalciferol in the liver and finally into 1, 25-dihydroxycholecalciferol in the kidney.

(D) Vitamin D is the active form of vitamin D3.

(5) Which of the following are mechanisms through which the kidneys control blood pressure?

(A) Intracellular volume regulation.

(B) Production of erythropoietin.

(C) Rennin-angiotensin-aldosterone system.

(D) Effect of prostaglandins.

(6) Which of these features describes the kidneys?

(A) The healthy adult kidneys are paired reddish-brown organs.

(B) Each kidney has about 1–1.3 million tubules.

(C) Each kidney has anterior and posterior surfaces, as well as medial and lateral margins.

(D) The kidneys are both about 1000 g.

(7) Which of the following is not true about the fascial coverings of the kidneys?

(A) The adipose capsule protects the kidneys from trauma and helps maintain the position of the kidneys within the abdominal cavity.

(B) The renal fascia provides structural support and attaches the kidney to the abdominal wall.

(C) The renal capsule maintains the kidney's structural integrity and shape and protects its tissue.

(D) The peritoneum maintains the kidney's structural integrity and shape and protects its tissue.

(8) Which is not true about the blood supply of the kidney?

(A) The kidneys receive their blood supply from the renal arteries.

(B) The blood vessels in the kidneys are extremely specialized to support the kidneys in urine formation.

(C) The kidneys receive about 25% of the cardiac output.

(D) Interlobular arteries give rise to efferent arterioles.

(9) Which of the following is not the arterial branch within the kidney?

(A) Segmental arteries.

(B) Interlobar arteries.

(C) Glomerular artery.

(D) Interlobular arteries.

(10) Which of the following is not true about the internal structure of the kidney?

(A) The kidney is composed of three layers: the cortex, medulla, and the renal sinus.

(B) It is dark and granular in appearance. It contains the renal corpuscles and convoluted tubules, which may extend into the inner medulla.

(C) The renal sinus is occupied by the renal pelvis, calices, blood vessels, nerves, and fat. These structures enter and exit the renal sinus through the hilum.

(D) The internal structure is made up of the renal fascia, the renal capsule, and the extra renal pad of fat.

(11) A 68-year-old patient with a history of diabetes and heart failure is admitted to the hospital for a hip replacement procedure. The patient is prescribed several medications as part of their perioperative care. During the hospital stay, the patient's creatinine levels begin to rise. What is the most likely factor that disrupted creatinine levels in this patient?

(A) Age over 60 years.

(B) Pre-existing renal insufficiency.

(C) Volume depletion.

(D) Perioperative care drugs.

(12) What is the initial step in the management of glomerulonephritis?

(A) Diet counseling.

(B) Regular renal function tests.

(C) Immunosuppressive drugs.

(D) Control blood pressure.

(13) A patient with glomerulonephritis presents with significant lower extremity swelling and high urinary output. You recognize that these symptoms are most indicative of which condition?

(A) Acute kidney injury.

(B) Chronic kidney disease.

(C) Nephrotic syndrome.

(D) Urinary tract infection.

(14) A nephrologist attempts to evaluate a patient with suspected glomerulonephritis. Despite clinical signs, the specific subtype of glomerulonephritis remains unclear. What diagnostic approach might the specialist consider?

(A) Do not attempt to identify the subtype.

(B) Assess for nephrotic syndrome.

(C) Perform a kidney biopsy.

(D) Order routine urine tests.

(15) A 40-year-old patient presents with acute kidney injury. The history reveals chronic contact with heavy metals through his work in a metal foundry. Which part of the kidney is most likely to be affected by the chronic inhalation of heavy metals?

(A) Glomeruli.

(B) Distal tubules.

(C) Proximal tubules.

(D) Loop of Henle.

(16) A 65-year-old patient with glomerulonephritis experiences difficulty breathing and high blood pressure. Which medication may be used to improve the patient's symptoms?

(A) Corticosteroids.

(B) Nitroprusside.

(C) Rituximab.

(D) Furosemide.

(17) When administering antibiotics to a patient with CKD and a GFR of 45 mL/min/1.73 m^2, why must the healthcare provider consider the patient's renal function?

(A) To determine the appropriate frequency of antibiotic administration.

(B) To assess the risk of allergic reactions to antibiotics.

(C) To evaluate the need for additional fluid intake with antibiotics.

(D) To check for potential interactions with antihypertensive medications.

(18) A 28-year-old patient presents with flank pain and blood in their urine. She reports a family history of polycystic kidney disease. When do the symptoms of polycystic kidney disease typically manifest in patients with this genetic condition?

(A) The first decade of life.

(B) The second decade of life.

(C) The third decade of life.

(D) The fourth decade of life.

(19) A female patient with a family history of Autosomal Dominant Polycystic Kidney presents with dysuria, flank pain, and fatigue. You recognize that the most likely cause of these symptoms is:

(A) UTI.

(B) Kidney stone.

(C) Worsening of ADPKD.

(D) Acute kidney injury.

(20) A 60-year-old patient with ADPKD discusses treatment options with their healthcare provider. By what age do a considerable portion of ADPKD patients require a kidney transplant?

(A) 40 years.

(B) 50 years.

(C) 60 years.

(D) 70 years.

(21) What is the primary purpose of using the Albumin-Creatinine Ratio (ACR) in the classification of chronic kidney disease?

(A) To estimate the glomerular filtration rate.

(B) To assess the severity of proteinuria.

(C) To evaluate electrolyte imbalances.

(D) To measure creatinine clearance.

(22) Which of the following ACR values is usually associated with normal kidney function?

(A) ACR of 2 mg/mmol.

(B) ACR of 20 mg/mmol.

(C) ACR of 200 mg/mmol.

(D) ACR of 2000 mg/mmol.

(23) A patient with an eGFR of 20 mL/min/1.73m^2 and an ACR of 20 mg/mmol belongs to which stage of CKD?

(A) CKD G4A2.

(B) CKD G5A3.

(C) CKD G2A1.

(D) CKD G2A2.

(24) When assessing CKD, the ACR classification is used alongside eGFR staging. What does the ACR classification specifically measure for a more comprehensive assessment of CKD?

(A) Albumin-to-Creatinine Ratio in urine.

(B) Acid-Base Balance in blood.

(C) Calcium-to-Phosphorus Ratio in blood.

(D) Anemia Count Ratio in blood.

(25) Which lifestyle changes are often recommended for individuals with stage 1 chronic kidney disease?

(A) No lifestyle changes are necessary at this stage.

(B) Increased salt intake.

(C) Smoking cessation and blood pressure control.

(D) Increased protein consumption.

(26) A 55-year-old man has an eGFR of 10 mL/min/1.73m^2 and experiences significant fatigue, body weakness, and fluid retention. Which of the following statements is not correct concerning this patient?

(A) The man is in stage 5 CKD.

(B) He will benefit from renal transplant.

(C) His management plan should be based on risk prevention and slowing disease progression.

(D) The fatigue and body weakness might be due to anemia.

(27) Which of the following is a characteristic clinical feature of stage 4 CKD?

(A) Normal eGFR.

(B) Severe kidney damage.

(C) Mild proteinuria.

(D) Presence of urinary incontinence.

(28) When evaluating a patient with CKD, the designation of Stage G3a A2 indicates which of the following conditions?

(A) Kidney function is moderately decreased with mild levels of albuminuria.

(B) Kidney function is severely decreased with high levels of albuminuria.

(C) Kidney function is mildly decreased with moderate levels of albuminuria.

(D) Kidney function is normal with severe levels of albuminuria.

(29) A patient being managed for CKD sustained a stress fracture of the femoral shaft. Which of the following provides the most likely explanation for the fracture?

(A) Osteoporosis from decreased activation of vitamin D.

(B) Metastasis from a possible renal tumor.

(C) Osteoporosis from decreased serum phosphate.

(D) Anemia.

(30) Which of the following is not a common manifestation of uremic symptoms in a patient with stage 4 CKD?

(A) Anemia.

(B) Mental dysfunction.

(C) Increased susceptibility to infection.

(D) Hypokalemia.

(31) It is important to be aware of nephrotoxic drugs that can further impair kidney function in patients with chronic kidney disease. Which of the following medications is commonly recognized as nephrotoxic?

(A) Acetaminophen.

(B) Amlodipine.

(C) NSAIDs.

(D) Levothyroxine.

(32) Which of these is a significant contributor to the increasing occurrence of AKI?

(A) The decreased use of nephrotoxic drugs.

(B) The decreased use of invasive procedures.

(C) An improved diagnostic acumen.

(D) The decreased aging population.

(33) Which of the below conditions is the most common cause of prerenal AKI?

(A) Acute tubular necrosis.

(B) Congestive cardiac failure.

(C) Nephrotoxic exposure.

(D) Acute glomerulonephritis.

(34) Which of the following is a characteristic of CKD often seen on renal ultrasound?

(A) Enlarged kidneys.

(B) The presence of cysts within the kidneys.

(C) Small and echogenic kidneys.

(D) Bilateral hydronephrosis.

(35) In CKD, what range of GFR is seen in stage five CKD (also known as ESKD)?

(A) GFR >90 mL/min/1.73m^2.

(B) GFR 60–89 mL/min/1.73m^2.

(C) GFR 30–59 mL/min/1.73m^2.

(D) GFR <15 ml/min/1.73m^2.

(36) Which class of medication should be used cautiously in CKD patients due to its potential nephrotoxic effects?

(A) Beta-blockers.

(B) Calcium channel blockers.

(C) NSAIDs.

(D) ACEIs.

(37) In CKD, what is the primary reason for the development of bone and mineral disorders?

(A) Decreased vitamin D intake.

(B) Altered calcium and phosphate balance.

(C) Excessive parathyroid hormone secretion.

(D) Reduced bone marrow function.

(38) Which of the following factors is not considered in the determination of AKI prognosis?

(A) The age of the patient.

(B) The duration of the illness.

(C) Blood pressure levels.

(D) The presence of proteinuria.

(39) Which of the following electrolyte imbalances is most commonly associated with advanced CKD?

(A) Hypernatremia.

(B) Hyperkalemia.

(C) Hypocalcemia.

(D) Hypophosphatemia.

(40) Which of the following is not a common cause of CKD?

(A) Diabetes mellitus.

(B) Hypertension.

(C) AKI.

(D) Glomerulonephritis.

(41) In kidney disease patients, high levels of fibroblast growth factor 23 (FGF23) are often associated with:

(A) High levels of phosphate.

(B) Low levels of phosphate.

(C) Normal levels of phosphate.

(D) No correlation with phosphate levels.

(42) Anemic patients with kidney disease are deficient in which of the following that is responsible for stimulating hematopoiesis?

(A) Thyroid hormone.

(B) Erythropoietin (EPO).

(C) Parathyroid hormone (PTH).

(D) Renin.

(43) What type of anemia is seen in kidney disease as a result of a hormone deficiency mentioned in the question above?

(A) Iron-deficiency anemia.

(B) Hemolytic anemia.

(C) Sickle cell anemia.

(D) Normocytic normochromic anemia.

(44) Ms. Cooper had anemia due to kidney disease. She was given iron supplements that improved her symptoms. Which subsequent treatment should be given to better correct the anemia?

(A) Erythropoiesis-stimulating agents (ESAs).

(B) Iron supplements.

(C) Nonsteroidal anti-inflammatory drugs (NSAIDs).

(D) Anticoagulants.

(45) The laboratory results for Joseph show accumulation of phosphate in the blood. This is secondary to his kidney disease and he currently has mineral and bone disorders. What term describes this finding?

(A) Hypokalemia.

(B) Hyperphosphatemia.

(C) Hypercalcemia.

(D) Hyponatremia.

(46) Eliana has experienced recurrent kidney stones, bone pain, and weakness. After the blood work, her lab results show low parathyroid hormone levels and high serum calcium levels. Which mineral and bone disorder associated with chronic kidney disease presents in this way?

(A) Hypoparathyroidism.

(B) Hyperparathyroidism.

(C) Renal osteodystrophy.

(D) Osteoarthritis.

(47) Mineral and bone disorders present complications in kidney subject patients at high risk of developing fractures due to weakened bones. Which of the following are you likely to suspect in such patients?

(A) Finger fractures.

(B) Hip fractures.

(C) Skull fractures.

(D) Rib fractures.

(48) Kidney disease patients are prone to one primary electrolyte imbalance. Which of the following represents this imbalance?

(A) Hypokalemia.

(B) Hypercalcemia.

(C) Hyperkalemia.

(D) Hyponatremia.

(49) While preparing to leave after a whole day of nursing duty, you hear Mr. Snow calling and complaining of some muscle weakness and cramps. You suspect he might even have cardiac arrhythmias. Which electrolyte imbalance would cause this?

(A) Hypokalemia.

(B) Hypernatremia.

(C) Hypocalcemia.

(D) Hyperkalemia.

(50) A 55-year-old came in complaining of some muscle weakness, rapid heartbeat, skipping heartbeats at times, as well as confusion. She is a patient with kidney disease. Which imbalance could cause these complaints?

(A) Hypokalemia.

(B) Hypophosphatemia.

(C) Hyperkalemia.

(D) Hypercalcemia.

(51) A patient on peritoneal dialysis for the past 6 months presents with abdominal pain and a fever of 12 hours duration. Physical examination shows he has a cloudy dialysate and a board-like abdomen. What is the most likely diagnosis?

(A) Appendicitis.

(B) Peritonitis.

(C) Large bowel obstruction.

(D) Acute pyelonephritis.

(52) Which of the following statements is true regarding peritoneal dialysis?

(A) Peritonitis is the most common complication.

(B) It requires a professional healthcare provider at all times.

(C) The organism causing dialysis-associated peritonitis should be isolated first before initiating treatment.

(D) It is preferred for emergency cases of dialysis.

(53) What is the main purpose of providing immunosuppressive therapy after a kidney transplant?

(A) To decrease the risk of infection.

(B) To decrease the chance of neoplastic transformation.

(C) To prevent rejection of the transplanted kidney.

(D) To decrease the risk of post-operation bleeding.

(54) What are the properties of substances like inulin or radiolabeled ethylenediamine-tetra-acetic acid (EDTA) that make them ideal for measuring GFR?

(A) They are not excreted through the kidney at all.

(B) They are completely filtered at the glomerulus and completely reabsorbed by the renal tubules.

(C) They are completely filtered at the glomerulus and significantly secreted by the renal tubules.

(D) They are completely filtered at the glomerulus and are neither secreted nor reabsorbed by the renal tubules.

(55) Which one of the following urine analysis parameters is normal?

(A) 4 WBC/HPF on microscopy.

(B) Urine output of 200ml over 24 hours.

(C) Positive nitrite and leukocyte esterase.

(D) +3 ketone on dipstick.

(56) An active hepatitis C infection is considered a relative contraindication for kidney transplant preparation, as it can impact post-transplant outcomes. What is the current recommendation regarding hepatitis C infection and kidney transplantation?

(A) Hepatitis C infection is an absolute contraindication for kidney transplantation.

(B) Hepatitis C infection should not be considered a contraindication for kidney transplantation.

(C) Hepatitis C infection is a relative contraindication for kidney transplantation.

(D) Hepatitis C infection is only a contraindication for kidney transplantation in certain cases.

(57) A 65-year-old patient with uncontrolled hypertension, uncontrolled diabetes, and who has been a chronic smoker for the last 10 years comes to the nursing station for a kidney biopsy. The nurse declines to go ahead with the procedure after a view of the patient's chart. What is the most likely reason for the refusal?

(A) His uncontrolled hypertension.

(B) His uncontrolled diabetes.

(C) His chronic smoking history.

(D) His age.

(58) A 67-year-old man undergoes a kidney biopsy. Two hours later, he complains of left flank pain. Which of the following is the most likely diagnosis?

(A) Pneumothorax.

(B) Retroperitoneal hematoma.

(C) Post-biopsy syndrome.

(D) Kidney infarction.

(59) Which of the following urine analysis results is suggestive of the glomerular origin of renal pathology for a 34-year-old male patient who presented with cola-colored urine and generalized body swelling?

(A) Dysmorphic RBC.

(B) Granular casts.

(C) Uniform shaped RBC.

(D) ccvvb casts.

(60) Which of the following events can falsely decrease the BUN level when it is used to assess kidney function?

(A) Dehydration.

(B) Malnutrition.

(C) Glucocorticoids.

(D) High protein diet.

(61) Which of these statements about short daily hemodialysis is false?

(A) There is better hemodynamic stability with short daily dialysis.

(B) Sessions are done thrice a week for a few hours.

(C) There is a better survival rate with short daily hemodialysis.

(D) Toxins are removed more effectively than the conventional type.

(62) Mrs. X is a 49-year-old woman diagnosed with ESRD. She needs hemodialysis. Which factors are important to consider to guide her decision for home or in-center dialysis?

(A) Her physical state.

(B) Her physical and mental state.

(C) Her ability to understand and administer treatment independently.

(D) All of the above.

(63) Which of the following best describes nocturnal dialysis?

(A) Sessions are done nightly.

(B) Sessions are shorter during the day every other night.

(C) Sessions are done between six to eight hours three or more days a week at night.

(D) Sessions can only be done at the hospital or dialysis center.

(64) The process by which excess fluid is removed from the blood during hemodialysis is called:

(A) Hemodialysis.

(B) Hemodiafiltration.

(C) Filtration.

(D) Ultrafiltration.

(65) Which of these are a disadvantage of home dialysis?

(A) Allows for a flexible schedule.

(B) Less expenditure on nursing staff.

(C) Improves the quality of life.

(D) Patients and their caregivers must be trained to operate and administer treatment safely.

(66) Classification of the types of hemodialysis based on the frequency of sessions includes all of the following except:

(A) Short daily hemodialysis.

(B) Conventional hemodialysis.

(C) In-center hemodialysis.

(D) Nocturnal hemodialysis.

(67) Which of these has a higher rate of cardiovascular complications?

(A) Conventional dialysis.

(B) Short daily dialysis.

(C) Nocturnal dialysis.

(D) Home nocturnal hemodialysis.

(68) During hemodialysis, through which semipermeable membrane does the solute travel?

(A) Plasma.

(B) Dialysate.

(C) Body fluid.

(D) None of the above.

(69) The dialysate serves as the region of higher concentration during hemodialysis. What is the reason for this?

(A) The dialysate has a high concentration of waste.

(B) The dialysate has a low concentration of waste.

(C) The dialysate has a high concentration of electrolytes.

(D) The dialysate has a low concentration of electrolytes.

(70) The following statements are true about in-center dialysis except:

(A) Treatment services are provided at home.

(B) Treatment is provided in the hospital or a specialized center.

(C) Treatment is more common than home hemodialysis.

(D) Treatment must be administered by the patient's relative or caregiver.

(71) Which of the following postoperative measures is inappropriate after AVF creation?

(A) Observe for signs of infection.

(B) Allow permissive hypotension for two weeks after AVF creation.

(C) Adequate pain management.

(D) Elevation of the limb after the procedure.

(72) Mr. Mark is a 57-year-old CKD patient who is being discharged after AVG creation. What should the discharging nurse tell Mr. Mark to help the long-term functionality of the AVG?

(A) Apply constrictive stockings over the operated arm.

(B) Apply warm compresses over the operated arm.

(C) Apply heavy loads over the operated arm.

(D) Avoid drug administration and procedures over the operated arm.

(73) What is the correct technique for needle placement during AVF cannulation?

(A) Position the arterial needle close to the anastomosis and the venous needle at least 5cm distal to the arterial needle, with the needle tip facing the heart.

(B) Position the venous needle close to the anastomosis and the arterial needle at least 5cm distal to the venous needle, with the needle tip facing the heart.

(C) Position the arterial needle close to the anastomosis and the venous needle at least 10cm distal to the arterial needle, with the needle tip facing the heart.

(D) Position the venous needle close to the anastomosis and the arterial needle at least 10cm distal to the venous needle, with the needle tip facing the heart.

(74) How can hypotension after AV fistula creation be prevented?

(A) Elevate the limbs.

(B) Increase dry weight.

(C) Cold compress to site.

(D) Avoid cannulation.

(75) Which of the following statements regarding patient education on central venous catheters is untrue?

(A) Do not submerge the catheter site in water.

(B) Use waterproof dressing before showering.

(C) Report pain and swelling over the catheter site urgently.

(D) Remove the caps when the catheters are not in use.

(76) Which of the following patients is the ideal candidate to start dialysis access planning?

(A) A CKD patient with a GFR of 50.

(B) A CKD patient with a GFR of 72.

(C) A CKD patient with a GFR of 26.

(D) A CKD patient with a GFR of 10.

(77) When assessing a patient for arteriovenous fistula (AVF) formation using duplex ultrasound, which combination of arterial and venous diameters is considered optimal?

(A) Artery diameter greater than 1.6mm and vein diameter greater than 2mm.

(B) Artery diameter greater than 2mm and vein diameter greater than 1.6mm.

(C) Artery diameter greater than 2.5mm and vein diameter greater than 3mm.

(D) Artery diameter greater than 1mm and vein diameter greater than 1.5mm.

(78) What is the best predictor for determining when to initiate hemodialysis in a patient with chronic kidney disease?

(A) The patient's blood pressure readings.

(B) The presence of uremic symptoms.

(C) The patient's dietary preferences.

(D) The level of physical activity of the patient.

(79) Which type of vascular access should be avoided in patients who may require permanent access later due to a greater risk of stenosis?

(A) Radiocephalic fistula.

(B) Radiobasilic fistula.

(C) Subclavian catheter.

(D) Femoral catheter.

(80) What type of cannulation technique has the highest risk of infection?

(A) Rope ladder.

(B) Buttonhole.

(C) Area puncture.

(D) They all have equal risk.

(81) Which of the following types of vascular access is most commonly used for long-term hemodialysis treatments?

(A) Peripheral intravenous catheter.

(B) Arteriovenous fistula (AVF).

(C) Central venous catheter (CVC).

(D) Arteriovenous graft (AVG).

(82) Which of the following statements is accurate in relation to how an AVF differs from an arteriovenous graft (AVG) for hemodialysis?

(A) AVFs are created surgically, while AVGs occur naturally.

(B) AVFs have a lower risk of infection than AVGs.

(C) AVFs require frequent needle insertions, while AVGs do not.

(D) AVFs are used for temporary access.

(83) Which of the following electrolyte imbalances is more likely to occur in patients on hemodialysis and may require supplementation during treatment?

(A) Hyponatremia.

(B) Hyperkalemia.

(C) Hypocalcemia.

(D) Hypophosphatemia.

(84) Where does ultrafiltration occur during the hemodialysis process?

(A) In the blood pump.

(B) In the arterial line.

(C) In the dialyzer.

(D) In the venous line.

(85) What drives the diffusion of small solutes across the dialyzer membrane during hemodialysis?

(A) Concentration gradients.

(B) Ultrafiltration.

(C) Dialysate pressure.

(D) Hemodynamic factors.

(86) Which of the following molecules is cleared less efficiently in hemodialysis due to its larger size?

(A) Urea.

(B) Creatinine.

(C) Sodium.

(D) Potassium.

(87) What is the primary purpose of ultrafiltration during hemodialysis?

(A) Removal of waste products.

(B) Enhancement of solute diffusion.

(C) Control of fluid balance.

(D) Prevention of membrane damage.

(88) What type of dialyzer allows for precise ultrafiltration control and is well-suited for reuse?

(A) Coil dialyzers.

(B) Parallel plate dialyzers.

(C) Hollow-fiber dialyzers.

(D) Synthetic dialyzers.

(89) What is a key feature of hollow-fiber dialyzers that distinguishes them from parallel plate dialyzers in hemodialysis?

(A) Lower anticoagulant requirements.

(B) Ability to handle a high volume of blood.

(C) Reduced efficiency in toxin removal.

(D) Smaller surface area for filtration.

(90) What type of dialyzer is commonly used in contemporary practice in the USA?

(A) Coil dialyzers.

(B) Parallel plate dialyzers.

(C) Hollow-fiber dialyzers.

(D) High-flux dialyzers.

(91) Which dialysis machine is preferred due to the type of membrane it utilizes?

(A) Parallel plate.

(B) Hollow fiber.

(C) Coil tube

(D) Hollow plate

(92) In cases of acute poisoning, under what circumstance is dialysis most commonly required?

(A) When the patient experiences a mild allergic reaction to the toxic substance.

(B) When the toxic substance is known to be dialyzable.

(C) When there is a delay in hospital admission after poisoning.

(D) When the patient has a history of chronic kidney disease.

(93) Of the below parameters, which require monitoring before and during dialysis?

(A) Blood pressure, pulse, temperature, flow rate and respiratory rate.

(B) Blood pressure, cough reflex, diabetes and pulse.

(C) Blood pressure, air pressure, temperature, flow rate and albumin level.

(D) Blood pressure, cough reflex, respiratory rate and flow rate.

(94) How might the mechanism of dialysis be explained to a patient?

(A) It works using adhesion.

(B) It utilizes reverse osmosis.

(C) It impacts capillary action.

(D) It works through cohesion.

(95) What combination of the following makes up dialysate?

(A) Sodium, potassium, iron, carbon.

(B) Sodium, potassium and iron.

(C) Magnesium, sodium and potassium.

(D) Carbon, magnesium and potassium.

(96) What complication can arise in a dialysis patient due to an inappropriate sodium level in the dialysate?

(A) Hyperglycemia.

(B) Muscle cramps.

(C) Hemolysis.

(D) Air embolism.

(97) Which factor is most likely to contribute to chronic low blood pressure during hemodialysis sessions?

(A) High sodium concentration in the dialysate.

(B) Low sodium concentration in the dialysate.

(C) The temperature of the dialysate.

(D) The flow rate of the dialysate.

(98) After hemodialysis, a sixty-five-year-old patient feels weak. He says he experienced persistent fatigue and weakness during and after other dialysis sessions as well. Which component of the dialysate requires review?

(A) Calcium.

(B) Sodium.

(C) Potassium.

(D) Glucose (dextrose).

(99) What dialysate component will address metabolic acidosis in a fifty-seven-year-old hemodialysis patient?

(A) Bicarbonate.

(B) Sodium.

(C) Calcium.

(D) Potassium.

(100) A thirty-four-year-old patient on hemodialysis is noticeably susceptible to high blood potassium levels. Which component of the dialysate should be changed to manage this condition adequately?

(A) Calcium.

(B) Bicarbonate.

(C) Sodium.

(D) Potassium.

(101) Which of the following is not a clinical feature of hypotension?

(A) Low blood pressure readings above 150 mmHg.

(B) Cold clammy extremities.

(C) Pallor.

(D) Dizziness.

(102) Which of the following is a general measure for hypotension management?

(A) Decreasing dialysate temperature.

(B) Putting the patient in Trendelenburg position.

(C) Infusion of 0.9% saline or 20% albumin.

(D) All of the above.

(103) What defines hypotension in hemodialysis?

(A) Blood pressure >140 mmHg.

(B) Decreased systolic blood pressure by >20–30 mmHg from pre-dialysis levels.

(C) Decrease in diastolic blood pressure <100 mmHg.

(D) All of the above.

(104) Which of the following does not cause or predispose to hypotension in hemodialysis?

(A) Hypernatremia.

(B) Autonomic dysfunction.

(C) Antibiotic medication.

(D) Dehydration.

(105) What is a set of neurologic and systemic symptoms that occur primarily due to cerebral edema in dialyzed patients?

(A) Air embolism.

(B) Dialysis disequilibrium syndrome.

(C) Dialyzer reaction.

(D) First-use syndrome.

(106) Which of the following can cause muscle cramps?

(A) Intravascular volume depletion.

(B) Hypertension.

(C) Rapid sodium removal.

(D) All except (B).

(107) Which of the following is not a common electrolyte disturbance in hemodialysis?

(A) Hypochloremia.

(B) Hypo/hypernatremia.

(C) Hypocalcemia.

(D) Hyperkalemia.

(108) Which of the following is a proposed theory in dialysis disequilibrium syndrome?

(A) A reversal of osmotic shift induced by urea removal.

(B) A fall in intracellular pH.

(C) Both A and B.

(D) None of the above.

(109) What is the appropriate line of action to be carried out in a patient having seizure while on hemodialysis?

(A) Do a cardiac massage.

(B) Terminate the procedure.

(C) Observe for spontaneous abortion of seizure.

(D) Continue hemodialysis but at a faster rate.

(110) Which of the following describes the symptoms of dialysis disequilibrium syndrome?

(A) They are self-limiting.

(B) They resolve within 3–6 months.

(C) They include cardiovascular, musculoskeletal, and genitor-urinary symptoms.

(D) All of the above.

(111) A 40-year-old patient on hemodialysis reports that he changed his job 4 times in the past 6 months. What psychosocial aspect is most likely responsible for this issue?

(A) Poor physical fitness and stamina.

(B) Trouble maintaining personal relationships.

(C) Seeking high-paying jobs.

(D) Strict dietary compliance.

(112) A 35-year-old patient is transitioning from peritoneal dialysis to hemodialysis and is anxious about the change. What psychological challenge is the patient likely to face in the next few weeks?

(A) Fear of surgery.

(B) Unfounded fear.

(C) Difficulty adapting to a new dialysis modality.

(D) Fear of dietary restrictions.

(113) What is the recommended approach to assess the mental health of hemodialysis patients?

(A) Pre-therapeutic counseling sessions.

(B) Referral to an outpatient psychiatry clinic.

(C) Screen measures for anxiety and depression.

(D) In-person interviews with a psychologist.

(114) What is the primary pharmacological treatment for depression in hemodialysis patients?

(A) Tricyclic antidepressants.

(B) Selective serotonin reuptake inhibitors (SSRIs).

(C) Selective norepinephrine reuptake inhibitors (SNRIs).

(D) Monoamine oxidase inhibitors.

(115) A 65-year-old patient on hemodialysis presents with signs of inflammation at the site where the dialysis catheter is inserted. The area is also swollen and has started to discharge pus. What is the most likely pathogen responsible for this infection?

(A) Escherichia coli.

(B) Staphylococcus aureus.

(C) Pseudomonas aeruginosa.

(D) Streptococcus pyogenes.

(116) A nurse in a hemodialysis unit is about to perform an aseptic procedure. What action should she take to lower the risk of microbial transmission during this procedure?

(A) Wear gloves.

(B) Use sterile clothing.

(C) Wash hands frequently.

(D) Use hand antiseptics.

(117) A nurse is responsible for handling various items introduced to a patient's dialysis station. She notices an ampoule of intravenous medication labeled for single use. What should the nurse do with this ampoule?

(A) Dispose of it directly after the session.

(B) Clean and disinfect it.

(C) Reuse it for another patient to preserve resources.

(D) Prepare medications in a designated area.

(118) In a busy hemodialysis unit, the staff is concerned about the potential for blood contamination. What practice is recommended to minimize this risk?

(A) Reuse external venous and arterial pressure transducer filters.

(B) Clean surfaces frequently touched by patients with water and a clean cloth.

(C) Proper disinfection of dialysis stations between patients.

(D) Avoid capping dialyzer ports and clamping tubing.

(119) An incident in a hemodialysis unit occurred where blood was spilled on the patient's station. Which disinfectant should be used for the area?

(A) A 1:1000 dilution of household bleach.

(B) A 1:10 dilution of household bleach.

(C) A 1:100 dilution of household bleach.

(D) A 1:10000 dilution of household bleach.

(120) A healthcare provider is about to perform a procedure that carries a risk of blood spatter during hemodialysis. What personal protective equipment should the provider wear to ensure safety?

(A) Surgical masks.

(B) Gowns.

(C) Hairnets.

(D) Sandals.

(121) In patients with chronic kidney disease, which underlying condition is a common reason for a lack of response to recombinant human erythropoietin treatment for anemia?

(A) Hypothyroidism.

(B) Diabetes.

(C) Hypertension.

(D) Asthma.

(122) A patient has candida infection following dialysis and was given fluconazole. Which of the following best describes the mechanism of action of this drug?

(A) It decreases ergosterol synthesis by interfering with cytochrome P450 activity, which inhibits cell membrane formation.

(B) It increases ergosterol synthesis by interfering with cytochrome P450 activity, which inhibits cell membrane formation.

(C) It decreases ergosterol synthesis by interfering with cytochrome P450 activity, which promotes cell membrane formation.

(D) It increases ergosterol synthesis by interfering with cytochrome P450 activity, which promotes cell membrane formation.

(123) A 42-year-old male was diagnosed with chronic kidney disease two years ago. He has been on regular dialysis, as indicated by the nephrology consultation. Now, he complains of easy fatigability. On general examination, pallor was noted, and on blood examination, he was found to have anemia. Recombinant human erythropoietin was prescribed for the patient. Which of the following best describes the mechanism of action of this prescribed drug?

(A) It increases the RBC lifespan.

(B) It induces erythropoiesis.

(C) It inhibits RBC destruction.

(D) It decreases the blood viscosity and hematocrit level.

(124) Which of the following best describes the chemical structure of heparin?

(A) It is a polymer of two sulfated disaccharide units: D-glucosamine-L-iduronic acid and D-glucosamine-D-glucuronic acid.

(B) It is a polymer of two sulfated disaccharide units: L-glucosamine-D-iduronic acid and L-glucosamine-L-glucuronic acid.

(C) It is a polymer of two sulfated disaccharide units: D-glucosamine-L-glucuronic acid and D-glucosamine-D-glucuronic acid.

(D) It is a polymer of two sulfated disaccharide units: D-glucosamine-L-glucuronic acid and D-glucosamine-D-iduronic acid.

(125) A 49-year-old male presented to the OPD with a complaint of fever and tachycardia following dialysis. He is a known case of chronic renal failure with a current creatinine clearance of 30 ml/min. A detailed blood investigation was done, and post-infection by streptococcus viridians was diagnosed. On sensitivity testing, it was found to be sensitive to gentamicin. Which of the following best describes the use of gentamicin in this patient?

(A) Only seventy percent of the daily dose is to be used.

(B) Only fifty percent of the daily dose is to be used.

(C) Only thirty percent of the daily dose is to be used.

(D) Only ten percent of the daily dose is to be used.

(126) Heparin is one of the most commonly used drugs during dialysis. Which statement best describes the mechanism of action of this drug?

(A) It acts directly by activating plasma antithrombin III.

(B) It acts indirectly by activating plasma antithrombin III.

(C) It acts by binding and depleting factor VIIa.

(D) It mainly inhibits the extrinsic pathway.

(127) A 49-year-old female with chronic kidney disease has undergone dialysis for the last seven months. Today, she was found to have acute hyperkalemia with a value of 7.5 mmol/l. Which of the following best describes the medical management for this patient?

(A) Intravenous administration of propofol.

(B) Intravenous administration of salbutamol.

(C) Intramuscular administration of adrenaline.

(D) Intramuscular administration of sorbitol.

(128) A 61-year-old male with chronic kidney disease has been on dialysis for the last three years. He had regular checkups, and his phosphate values were found to be at the higher limit. Which drug is best implicated to prevent and treat hyperphosphatemia in this patient?

(A) Calcium-containing phosphate binders.

(B) Aluminum-containing phosphate binders.

(C) Sodium-containing phosphate binders.

(D) Magnesium-containing phosphate binders.

(129) A 42-year-old female with chronic kidney disease was prescribed calcitriol. Which statement best justifies the reason for the use of this drug?

(A) Kidneys convert Vitamin D to its active form, which is affected in chronic kidney conditions.

(B) Kidneys synthesize Vitamin D to its active form, which is affected in chronic kidney conditions.

(C) Kidneys metabolize Vitamin D to its active form, which is affected in chronic kidney conditions.

(D) Kidneys convert Vitamin D to its inactive form, which is affected in chronic kidney conditions.

(130) Cinacalcet is one of the most commonly prescribed drugs during dialysis. Which of the following best describes the indication for which the drug is given?

(A) Hyperthyroidism.

(B) Hyperparathyroidism.

(C) Hypothyroidism.

(D) Hypoparathyroidism.

(131) For which vaccines, when administered to kidney transplant patients, is it necessary to monitor serum levels?

(A) Anti-HCV vaccine.

(B) Anti-HBV vaccine.

(C) Anti-VZV vaccine.

(D) Anti-rabies vaccine.

(132) Which one of the following electrolyte abnormalities is associated with sirolimus?

(A) Hypercalcemia.

(B) Hyperkalemia.

(C) Hypokalemia.

(D) Hyperphosphatemia.

(133) Which of the following is not usually a side effect of cyclosporine when patients undergo treatment?

(A) Hypertension.

(B) Hyperchloremia.

(C) Gingival hyperplasia.

(D) Hirsutism.

(134) A 45-year-old female patient on her fifth post-transplant day complained of decreased urine amount and reddish discoloration of urine for one day associated with right lower quadrant abdominal pain. Subsequently, an abdominal ultrasound with a Doppler study was done. It revealed an enlarged kidney with absent flow in the renal vein. What is the best next step in the management of this patient?

(A) Contrast-enhanced CT scan.

(B) MR venography.

(C) Immediate surgery.

(D) Interventional radiology consultation.

(135) A 60-year-old female patient presented with an absent urine output of 12 hours duration. In addition, the patient has had reddish discoloration of urine since two days prior to presentation. Abdominal ultrasound showed a full urinary bladder with a normal-sized renal pelvis. Despite irrigating the catheter with saline, the urine output did not improve. What is the appropriate next step in the management of this patient?

(A) Nephrostomy tube insertion.

(B) Trial with $\alpha 1$ receptor blockers.

(C) Intermittent catheterization.

(D) Ureteral stent.

(136) Which of the following renal diseases could recur after transplantation?

(A) Focal segmental glomerular sclerosis.

(B) Polycystic kidney disease.

(C) Lipoid nephrosis.

(D) Tubulointerstitial nephritis.

(137) A 63-year-old male patient in his third post-transplant month presented with a productive cough of 3 weeks duration associated with fever, night sweats, and weight loss. The physical examination was unremarkable, and the chest x-ray revealed an upper lobe cavitation with hilar lymphadenopathy. What is the best next step in the management of this patient?

(A) Tuberculin skin test.

(B) Sputum gene X-pert.

(C) RHZE for two months, then RH for ten months.

(D) RHZE for two months, then RHZ for ten months.

(138) Which anti-TB drug should replace rifampicin if you fear drug interaction with immunosuppressive medications like cyclosporine?

(A) Amikacin.

(B) Ethionamide.

(C) Rifabutin.

(D) Capreomycin.

(139) A 50-year-old female patient, two months post-transplant, reported experiencing shortness of breath at rest for the past four days. She also reported having a low-grade fever intermittently, mild retrosternal pleuritic-type chest pain, and a dry cough over the past two weeks. Upon physical examination, her vital signs read as follows: BP: 100/70 mmHg, PR: 110 BPM, RR: 26 BPM, T: 100°F, and SpO2: 88%. During the examination of her respiratory system, no abnormalities were found. Air entry was sufficient and equal on both sides, with no additional sounds. A chest x-ray showed bilateral interstitial infiltrates in the middle and lower lobes. Which investigative modality would provide a high yield for confirming this diagnosis?

(A) Bronchoalveolar lavage.

(B) Chest CT scan.

(C) Induced sputum.

(D) LDH level and arterial blood gas analyses.

(140) Which of the following parameters warrant using corticosteroids in the above patient?

(A) PaO_2 greater than 70 mmHg.

(B) SpO_2 less than 88%.

(C) Pneumatocele on chest radiograph.

(D) Alveolar gradient greater than 35 mmHg.

(141) In a dialysis facility, a technician encounters disposable items that are contaminated with blood at the station of a 65-year-old patient. What is the recommended action to prevent contamination?

(A) Recycle them.

(B) Dispose of them in regular trash bags.

(C) Place them in designated bags.

(D) Reuse them if they can be sterilized.

(142) A 50-year-old patient with a history of diabetes and ESRD that requires hemodialysis presents with fever, elevated C-reactive protein (CRP), and nonspecific inflammatory signs. She states that she did not get vaccinated for hepatitis B. After a few tests, her healthcare provider decides to isolate this patient. Which of the following factors justifies the isolation of this patient?

(A) Vague symptoms of inflammation.

(B) A confirmed infection.

(C) A history of diabetes.

(D) Absence of hepatitis B vaccine.

(143) A 60-year-old patient on hemodialysis has a catheter for vascular access. The healthcare provider regularly examines the catheter exit site for signs of infection. What is the main purpose of this practice?

(A) Monitor patient comfort.

(B) Maintain catheter sterility.

(C) Look for leaks at the exit site.

(D) Ensure proper medication administration.

(144) A 59-year-old female with a chronic kidney disease has been on dialysis for the last three years and takes heparin. She presents with a fracture on the distal radius two cm above the wrist joint at the corticocancellous junction. An X-ray was done, and Colle's fracture was noted. On further investigation, she mentioned she had bone pain for the last eight months. Which of the following might be the best possible reason for this clinical presentation?

(A) Osteosarcoma as its risk increases due to long-term heparin use.

(B) Osteoarthritis as its risk increases due to long-term heparin use.

(C) Osteophytes as its risk increases due to long-term heparin use.

(D) Osteoporosis as its risk increases due to long-term heparin use.

(145) A 49-year-old female presents to the OPD with fatigue, muscle weakness, and body aches. A detailed investigation was done, and she was found to have secondary hyperparathyroidism, as she has had a known case of chronic kidney disease for the last three years. Which of the following is the best medical management for this case?

(A) Calcitriol.

(B) Cinacalcet.

(C) Erythropoietin.

(D) Angiotensin-converting enzyme.

(146) Which vaccine should not be given to kidney transplant patients?

(A) Influenza vaccine.

(B) Varicella vaccine.

(C) Pneumococcal vaccine.

(D) Meningococcal vaccine.

(147) A 50-year-old male patient, currently in his fifth month post-transplantation, recently experienced a dog bite incident. He reached the emergency department within half an hour of the occurrence. In the case of this individual, what are the guidelines or recommendations about administering a rabies vaccination?

(A) It should not be given since it is a live vaccine.

(B) It should not be given since the patient is in a period of intense immune suppression.

(C) It should be given because the rabies vaccine is safe for immunosuppressed patients.

(D) It should not be given because it has been associated with graft rejection.

(148) The serum creatinine of a 37-year-old female patient was monitored, and it was found to decrease by 0.3 mg/dl every 24 hours. Her serum electrolytes are normal. How should this patient be managed?

(A) Dialyses.

(B) Diuresis.

(C) Replacement fluid therapy.

(D) No additional intervention is required.

(149) A 43-year-old male patient on his first transplant month complained of frequency, urgency, and dysuria for five days. There was no pertinent positive finding on physical examination. Urinalysis showed 10-20 WBCs per high power field, with few bacteria and a positive leukocyte esterase. What is the best next step in the management of this patient?

(A) Ciprofloxacin 250 mg PO daily for 14 days.

(B) Urine culture.

(C) Fluconazole 200 mg PO daily for 14 days.

(D) Augmentin 500 mg PO BID for ten days.

(150) Which of the following conditions is an indication for renal biopsy after kidney transplantation?

(A) Slowly recovering renal function.

(B) New onset proteinuria.

(C) Renal artery stenosis.

(D) Refractory post-transplantation hypertension.

Test 2 Answers and Explanations

(1) (D) Sodium bicarbonate dissociates into sodium and bicarbonate, where the bicarbonate forms carbonic acid after combining with hydrogen.

Bicarbonate usually exists as sodium bicarbonate in the renal filtrate and is reabsorbed actively in the form of carbon dioxide from the proximal convoluted tubule. After dissociation of sodium bicarbonate into sodium and bicarbonate, the bicarbonate forms into carbonic acid after combining with hydrogen, which dissociates into carbon dioxide and water that enters the tubular cell.

(2) (D) It excretes unwanted waste products such as urea, uric acid, creatinine, and bilirubin, as well as other substances such as drugs and toxins.

The kidneys secrete hormones such as erythropoietin, thrombopoietin, and renin. It excretes unwanted waste products generated during metabolic activities in the body, such as urea, uric acid, creatinine, and bilirubin, as well as other substances such as drugs and toxins. It also produces vitamin D, which is essential for the absorption of calcium from the intestines.

(3) (D) Creatinine from muscle tissue.

The kidneys excrete the unwanted waste products, which are formed during metabolic activities in the body. This includes urea, which is generated from amino acid metabolism, uric acid from metabolism of nucleic acid, creatinine from metabolism of muscle tissue, bilirubin from the degradation of hemoglobin, and other substances such as drugs and toxins.

(4) (D) Vitamin D is the active form of vitamin D3.

The kidneys produce vitamin D, which is essential for the absorption of calcium from the intestines by converting vitamin D to its active form. Vitamin D3 is an active and important form of vitamin D. It is synthesized in the skin from 7-dehydrocholesterol by ultraviolet rays from the sunlight, which is then converted into 25-hydroxycholecalciferol in the liver and finally into 1, 25-dihydroxycholecalciferol in the kidney.

(5) (C) Rennin-angiotensin-aldosterone system.

Blood pressure regulation is achieved through the rennin-angiotensin-aldosterone system and by extracellular fluid volume regulation. The renin-angiotensin-aldosterone system (RAAS) is a complex hormonal cascade that helps control blood pressure and maintain the body's fluid and electrolyte balance. It is composed of renin, angiotensin, and aldosterone.

(6) (A) The healthy adult kidneys are paired reddish-brown organs.

The healthy adult kidneys are paired reddish-brown organs. Each kidney has anterior and posterior surfaces, medial and lateral margins, and superior and inferior poles.

(7) (D) The peritoneum maintains the kidney's structural integrity and shape and protects its tissue.

Each kidney is surrounded by three main layers: the renal fascia, the adipose capsule, and the renal capsule from the outer to the inner layers. The renal capsule provides structural support and attaches the kidney to the abdominal wall. The adipose capsule protects the kidneys from trauma and helps maintain the position of the kidneys within the abdominal cavity. The renal capsule maintains the kidney's structural integrity and shape and protects its tissue.

(8) (D) Interlobular arteries give rise to efferent arterioles.

The kidneys receive their blood supply from the renal arteries, which are branches of the abdominal aorta. The blood vessels in the kidneys are extremely specialized to support the kidneys in urine formation. Both kidneys receive about 25% of the cardiac output.

The arcuate artery subdivides into interlobular arteries, from which afferent arterioles arise.

(9) (C) Glomerular artery.

The kidneys receive their blood supply from the renal arteries, which are branches of the abdominal aorta. The renal artery divides into many segmental arteries after entering the kidney through the hilum, which gives rise to segmental arteries. The segmental artery further subdivides into interlobar arteries, which pass into the medulla between the medullary pyramids to form the arcuate arteries.

(10) (D) The internal structure is made up of the renal fascia, the renal capsule, and the extra renal pad of fat.

The kidney is composed of three layers: the cortex, medulla, and the renal sinus. It is dark and granular in appearance. It contains the renal corpuscles and convoluted tubules, which may extend into the inner medulla. The renal sinus is occupied by the renal pelvis, calices, blood vessels, nerves, and fat. These structures enter and exit the renal sinus through the hilum.

(11) (D) Perioperative care drugs.

This patient has multiple risk factors for drug-induced nephrotoxicity, which include age over 60, pre-existing renal insufficiency, volume depletion, and underlying medical conditions, such as diabetes and heart failure. These factors increase the vulnerability to kidney injury when exposed to certain medications.

(12) (D) Control blood pressure.

The main focus of management in glomerulonephritis is to control blood pressure. Although other aspects of management, such as diet counseling, regular renal function tests, and immunosuppressive drugs are important, blood pressure control is prioritized due to its impact on disease progression.

(13) (C) Nephrotic syndrome.

Nephrotic syndrome is characterized by a group of symptoms including significant proteinuria, hypoalbuminemia, and edema, especially in the lower extremities. High urinary output may not be a classic symptom of nephrotic syndrome, but it can occur in some cases. Given that the patient has glomerulonephritis, which is an inflammation of the glomeruli in the kidneys and can cause nephrotic syndrome, the presentation of significant swelling and changes in urinary output strongly suggests nephrotic syndrome.

(14) (C) Perform a kidney biopsy.

When the specific subtype of glomerulonephritis remains unclear, the gold standard procedure is to perform a kidney biopsy.

Sole reliance on clinical signs and symptoms may not provide a definitive diagnosis. Assessment of nephrotic syndrome is not effective to differentiate between GN subtypes. Routine urine tests are not useful.

(15) (C) Proximal tubules.

Chronic inhalation exposure to heavy metals, especially through occupational exposure, can affect the proximal tubules of the kidneys. This is essentially due to the reabsorption of ionized heavy metals in this region. Chronic exposure can cause the release of ionized heavy metals into the bloodstream, which contributes to low-grade inflammation, fibrosis, and kidney damage. Other parts of the kidney, such as the glomeruli, distal tubules, and loop of Henle, are less commonly involved in chronic heavy metal toxicity.

(16) (D) Furosemide.

Furosemide is a medication commonly used to help remove fluids and correct blood hypertension in patients with glomerulonephritis. The patient in this stem presents with pulmonary edema and lower extremity swelling. These symptoms are greatly relieved by loop diuretics.

Even though corticosteroids, nitroprusside, and rituximab may have other roles in managing glomerulonephritis, they are not typically used for fluid removal and blood pressure correction.

(17) (A) To determine the appropriate frequency of antibiotic administration.

For patients with CKD, particularly those with a reduced GFR like 45 mL/min/1.73 m^2, the renal function significantly affects how the body processes medications, including antibiotics. The kidneys play a vital role in filtering and eliminating many drugs from the body. In CKD, this function is impaired, which can cause the accumulation of drugs in the body and increase the risk of toxicity.

(18) (C) The third decade of life.

The symptoms of polycystic kidney disease manifest in patients in the third decade of life. Genetic counseling may be useful for couples with ADPKD.

(19) (A) UTI.

In a patient with a family history of Autosomal Dominant Polycystic Kidney Disease, the presence of dysuria (pain or discomfort during urination), flank pain, and fatigue are commonly indicative of a urinary tract infection. Patients with ADPKD are at a higher risk for UTIs due to the structural abnormalities in the kidneys that can be associated with this disease. The cysts common in ADPKD can obstruct urine flow and create an environment that is more susceptible to infections.

(20) (C) 60 years.

About half of the patients with ADPKD require a kidney transplant by the age of 60 years. Note that the age may vary among individuals.

(21) (B) To assess the severity of proteinuria.

ACR is based on the severity of proteinuria in the form of urinary albumin levels. ACR and urinary albumin excretion over 24 hours can classify CKD as follows:

- A1: ACR less than 3 mg/mmol or albumin excretion less than 30 mg/24hr.
- A2: ACR 3-30 mg/mmol or albumin excretion 30-300 mg/24hr.
- A3: ACR greater than 30 mg/mmol or albumin excretion greater than 300 mg/24hr.

(22) (A) ACR of 2 mg/mmol.

Albumin detected in the urine may represent a sign of kidney disease. The albumin-to-creatinine ratio (ACR) is most frequently applied to diagnose albuminuria. In spot urine specimens, the normal level of ACR is less than 3 mg/mmol.

(23) (A) CKD G4A2.

The stages of CKD are classified according to the eGFR as follows:

- Stage 1: Kidney damage with normal or increased eGFR.
- Stage 2: Mild reduction in eGFR.
- Stage 3a: Moderate reduction in eGFR.
- Stage 3b: Moderate reduction in eGFR.
- Stage 4: Severe reduction in eGFR.
- Stage 5: Kidney failure.

ACR and urinary albumin excretion over 24 hours can be used to classify CKD as follows:

- A1: ACR less than 3 mg/mmol or albumin excretion less than 30 mg/24hr.
- A2: ACR 3-30 mg/mmol or albumin excretion 30-300 mg/24hr.
- A3: ACR greater than 30 mg/mmol or albumin excretion greater than 300 mg/24hr.

(24) (A) Albumin-to-Creatinine Ratio in urine.

The ACR measures the amount of albumin relative to creatinine in the urine. This ratio is an important indicator of kidney damage and is used in the assessment and staging of CKD. A higher ACR indicates more significant kidney damage, as healthy kidneys usually do not allow a significant amount of albumin to pass into the urine. When used in conjunction with the estimated Glomerular Filtration Rate (eGFR), which measures kidney function, the ACR provides a more comprehensive understanding of a patient's CKD status.

(25) (C) Smoking cessation and blood pressure control.

In stage 1 CKD, early detection and management of kidney disease can help prevent further progression and complications. Patients with stage 1 CKD should work closely with their healthcare providers to address underlying risk factors and etiologies such as hypertension and smoking.

(26) (C) His management plan should be based on risk prevention and slowing disease progression.

Patients with stage 5 CKD usually require either hemodialysis, peritoneal dialysis or a kidney transplant to survive. Managing ESRD is essential for maintenance of life. Patients with stage 5 CKD often require comprehensive care from nephrologists and other healthcare providers.

(27) (B) Severe kidney damage.

Stage 4 chronic kidney disease represents a severe reduction in renal function, with a glomerular filtration rate between 15-29 mL/min/1.73m^2.

(28) (A) Kidney function is moderately decreased with mild levels of albuminuria.

"G3a" refers to a moderately decreased GFR, specifically in the range of 45-59 mL/min/1.73 m^2. This stage indicates a reduction in kidney function but not severely so. The "A2" designation refers to the level of albuminuria (protein in the urine), where A2 indicates a mild to moderate increase. Albuminuria is categorized based on the albumin-to-creatinine ratio, and A2 usually corresponds to an ACR of 30-300 mg/g, which indicates a moderate level of albuminuria.

(29) (A) Osteoporosis from decreased activation of vitamin D.

Osteoporosis in chronic kidney disease can be attributed to the following:

- Abnormal metabolism of calcium, phosphate, vitamin D, and parathyroid hormone.
- Calcification of soft tissue.
- Abnormal bone turnover and mineralization.

Decreased vitamin D activation due to failure of 1-alpha hydroxylation causes hypocalcemia, which invariably causes osteoporosis.

(30) (D) Hypokalemia.

Uremia is a clinical condition characterized by elevated serum concentrations of urea. It is a common feature in the advanced stages of CKD. Spontaneous bleeding can occur with severe uremia and may include gastrointestinal bleeding and anemia. Metabolic derangements such as hyperkalemia, metabolic acidosis, and hypocalcemia are also commonly seen in uremia. Uremic encephalopathy and increased susceptibility to infections are other common features seen.

(31) (C) NSAIDs.

Nonsteroidal anti-inflammatory drugs are well-known for their nephrotoxic potential, particularly in patients who may have existing kidney impairment like CKD. NSAIDs can reduce blood flow to the kidneys, which can exacerbate existing kidney problems or even cause acute kidney injury in susceptible individuals. They can also affect the levels of various electrolytes and disrupt kidney function.

(32) (C) An improved diagnostic acumen.

Improved diagnostic acumen and methods have enabled healthcare professionals to detect AKI in its initial stages, sometimes even before the occurrence of symptoms. This early detection has contributed to the increased occurrence of AKI, as individuals who might have been missed in previous years can now be diagnosed. This allows for timely intervention and prevents the condition from progressing.

(33) (B) Congestive cardiac failure.

Prerenal AKI is mainly caused by factors that cause reduced blood flow to the kidneys without structural impairment or damage to the renal tissues. One common cause is congestive cardiac failure, which can result in decreased blood perfusion to the kidneys.

(34) (C) Small and echogenic kidneys.

CKD is often associated with structural damage and changes in the kidneys. On renal ultrasound, CKD is characterized by small and echogenic (increased reflectivity) kidneys, which indicates ongoing and progressive damage to the renal tissue.

(35) (D) GFR <15 mL/min/1.73m^2.

The GFR is a measure of kidney function. It quantifies the rate at which the kidneys filter blood. A normal GFR is above 90 mL/min/1.73m^2. In stage five CKD, the GFR is <15 mL/min/1.73m^2. With such a low GFR, the kidneys can no longer carry out their excretory function, and waste products, toxins, and excess fluids build up in the blood.

In this scenario, renal replacement therapy in the form of dialysis or kidney transplant becomes necessary.

(36) (C) NSAIDs.

NSAIDs can impair blood flow to the kidneys and increase the risk of kidney damage, especially in patients with preexisting CKD. These drugs should be used cautiously, if at all, for individuals with compromised kidney function.

(37) (B) Altered calcium and phosphate balance.

The kidney plays a role in maintaining the balance of minerals in the body, particularly calcium and phosphate. In CKD, as kidney function declines, these balances are not maintained effectively, which causes dysfunction in calcium and phosphate metabolism that results in bone and mineral disorders.

(38) (D) The presence of proteinuria.

Proteinuria is not typically a factor considered in the determination of the prognosis of acute kidney injury (AKI). Proteinuria is more commonly associated with chronic kidney conditions rather than acute ones. The prognosis of AKI usually depends on factors such as the patient's age, the cause and duration of the kidney injury, the severity of the injury, and the patient's overall health status, including blood pressure levels.

(39) (B) Hyperkalemia.

In patients with advanced CKD, the kidneys struggle to excrete potassium, which results in its accumulation in the blood. The resultant effect is hyperkalemia. Other electrolyte disorders like hypernatremia are more commonly seen in conditions associated with dehydration. Hypocalcemia and hypophosphatemia are less common in cases of advanced CKD.

(40) (C) AKI.

AKI is a sudden and often reversible decline in kidney function. Isolated cases are not a common cause of CKD as they are often reversible. Repeated episodes of AKI can contribute to the development of CKD. Diabetes mellitus, hypertension, and glomerulonephritis are well-known causes of CKD.

(41) B) Low levels of phosphate.

In chronic kidney disease, elevated levels of FGF23 are associated with low levels of phosphate. FGF23 is a hormone that regulates phosphorus metabolism, and its levels increase in CKD as a compensatory mechanism to maintain normal serum phosphate levels in the setting of reduced renal capacity for phosphate excretion. FGF23 acts on the kidney to decrease phosphate reabsorption, which causes a reduced serum phosphate concentration.

(42) (B) Erythropoietin (EPO).

Erythropoietin (EPO) is a hormone produced by the kidney to stimulate hematopoiesis. In kidney disease, the hormone is inadequately produced which results in anemia.

(43) (D) Normocytic normochromic anemia.

Normocytic normochromic anemia is seen in kidney disease and results from deficient erythropoietin, toxic effects, or uremia in the bone marrow.

(44) (A) Erythropoiesis-stimulating agents (ESAs).

Since the deficiency of iron and anemia were corrected, then recombinant erythropoietin is given because it is more effective to correct and improve anemia and symptoms in kidney disease.

(45) (B) Hyperphosphatemia.

Loss of phosphorus homeostasis due to excretory failure in kidney disease patients results in positive balance hyperphosphatemia. This increases the concentration in the exchangeable phosphorus pool, often when the pool is reduced in size as in adynamic bone disease.

(46) (B) Hyperparathyroidism.

Primary hyperparathyroidism is characterized by raised serum calcium levels and low PTH levels. These findings can lead to bone pain.

(47) (B) Hip fractures.

Because the femur is a weight bearing bone, it can be weakened by the complications of mineral and bone disorders. The hip might fracture easily due to the weight of the patient.

(48) (C) Hyperkalemia.

Hyperkalemia is an electrolyte that is mostly affected in cases of imbalance due to impaired excretion of kidney disease. A patient can present with generalized fatigue, palpitations, muscle weakness, and parathesis.

(49) (A) Hypokalemia.

Potassium is required for the proper contraction of muscles as well conduction of electrical impulses. Its low levels disrupt these activities as evidenced by muscle weakness, cramps, and cardiac arrhythmias.

(50) (C) Hyperkalemia.

The symptoms are related to potassium imbalance in this patient.

(51) (B) Peritonitis.

Peritonitis is the most common complication associated with peritoneal dialysis. It results from an infection of the peritoneal cavity. Patients will often present with abdominal pain with cloudy dialysate and fever.

(52) (A) Peritonitis is the most common complication.

Peritoneal dialysis is a type of dialysis that involves use of the patient's peritoneal membrane as the partially permeable membrane. It is often reserved for chronic cases and has a limited role during emergency conditions. Additionally, peritoneal dialysis can be done at home by the patient or caregiver and does not require a machine. The most common complication associated with it is peritonitis. Treatment should be initiated empirically upon clinical suspicion.

(53) (C) To prevent rejection of the transplanted kidney.

Following transplant surgery, patients will need to take immunosuppressive therapy with the main aim of preventing graft rejection.

(54) (D) They are completely filtered at the glomerulus and are neither secreted nor reabsorbed by the renal tubules.

Substances like inulin or radiolabeled ethylenediamine-tetra-acetic acid (EDTA) are ideal to measure GFR because they are completely filtered at the glomerulus and are neither secreted nor reabsorbed by the renal tubules.

(55) (A) 4 WBC/HPF on microscopy.

On microscopic examination of a urine sample, the WBC count is said to be abnormal if the finding is ≥5WBC/HPF in males and ≥10WBC/HPF in women.

(56) (B) Hepatitis C infection should not be considered a contraindication for kidney transplantation.

The current recommendation is that hepatitis C infection should not be considered a contraindication for kidney transplantation. Studies and guidelines support this recommendation, and indicate that kidney transplant recipients with HCV infection can undergo transplantation, and that HCV infection should not be a barrier to kidney transplantation.

(57) (A) His uncontrolled hypertension.

Before a renal biopsy, it is important to control blood pressure and perform a complete blood count and coagulation profile. This is essential to decrease the risk of post-procedure bleeding.

(58) (B) Retroperitoneal hematoma.

Flank pain within hours of kidney biopsy suggests bleeding, likely into the perinephric space. This causes a retroperitoneal hematoma and is the most concerning complication.

(59) (A) Dysmorphic RBC.

RBC that originates in the glomerulus is dysmorphic. It is uniformly shaped if it originates from the lower structures of the nephron.

(60) (B) Malnutrition.

BUN levels increase in cases of dehydration, catabolic state, high protein diet, and drugs like glucocorticoids. On the other hand, BUN levels decrease in liver disease, malnutrition, old age, and SIADH.

(61) (B) Sessions are done thrice a week for a few hours.

The statement is false. The point of short daily dialysis is to have as close to normal kidney function as possible. Frequent sessions that last only a few hours are held to achieve this.

(62) (D) All of the above.

All the options are important factors that should guide Mrs. X in choosing.

(63) (C) Sessions are done between six to eight hours three or more days a week at night.

This statement best describes nocturnal dialysis. It mentioned the duration and frequency of the procedure.

(64) (D) Ultrafiltration.

Ultrafiltration is the process by which excess fluid is removed from the blood during hemodialysis.

(65) (D) Patients and their caregivers must be trained to operate and administer treatment safely.

Training patients and their caregivers requires much time, energy, effort, and commitment. The process may be tedious for both the healthcare professional and the patient. Some people may prefer care in a medical facility rather than at home, as healthcare professionals can attend to them in a more controlled environment.

(66) (C) In-center hemodialysis.

In-center hemodialysis is classified based on the location in which the procedure is carried out. It can be either at home or in a hospital or dialysis center.

(67) (A) Conventional hemodialysis.

Conventional hemodialysis is associated with an increased risk of cardiovascular complications.

(68) (B) Dialysate.

The toxins and excess fluid are filtered from the blood into the dialysis fluid, the dialysate.

(69) (B) The dialysate has a low concentration of waste.

During hemodialysis, the dialysate serves as the region of higher concentration for waste products. In the blood of the hemodialysis patient, there is a high concentration of waste. This concentration gradient allows for the diffusion of waste products from the blood into the dialysate across the semipermeable membrane of the dialyzer, and facilitates the removal of waste products from the patient's blood.

(70) (A) Treatment services are provided at home.

This statement is false. In-center dialysis is done at the hospital or a specialized dialysis center where medical and nursing staff carry out the process for the patient. All the other options are valid for in-center dialysis.

(71) (B) Allow permissive hypotension for two weeks after AVF creation.

Hypotension increases the risk of thrombosis formation, so increasing the dry weight for the first 2-4 weeks after AVF/AVG creation is important.

(72) (D) Avoid drug administration and procedures over the operated arm.

Patient education is one of the cornerstones for maintaining the functionality and health of the AVF/AVG. Patients should regularly check for thrill or bruit and avoid constrictive clothing, heavy loads on the affected arm, and extreme temperatures. They should also avoid allowing anyone to perform procedures or administer drugs in the access arm.

(73) (A) Position the arterial needle close to the anastomosis and the venous needle at least 5cm distal to the arterial needle, with the needle tip facing the heart.

Proper needle placement during dialysis involves situating the arterial needle nearest to the anastomosis from the surgical site. The venous needle should be positioned at least 5 cm away from the arterial needle, angled in the direction of venous flow toward the heart.

(74) (B) Increase dry weight.

Increasing the dry weight for 2-4 weeks after AV fistula creation can help prevent hypotension.

(75) (D) Remove the caps when the catheters are not in use.

Patients should ensure that clamps are closed, and caps are in place when the catheter is not in use to prevent potential complications such as bleeding and infection.

(76) (C) A CKD patient with a GFR of 26.

Dialysis access planning should start in CKD stage IV when education about CKD and modalities of renal replacement therapy should be discussed. From the available options, patient C has stage IV CKD (GFR of 15-29).

(77) (A) Artery diameter greater than 1.6mm and vein diameter greater than 2mm.

For successful arteriovenous fistula formation, it is important to ensure that the blood vessels used are of adequate size to support the fistula. Duplex ultrasound is commonly used to measure the diameters of the vessels. The optimal measurements for AVF formation are an artery diameter greater than 1.6mm and a vein diameter greater than 2mm. These dimensions are considered sufficient to provide adequate blood flow and reduce the risk of complications such as thrombosis or failure of the fistula.

(78) (B) The presence of uremic symptoms.

The best predictor for the initiation of hemodialysis in patients with chronic kidney disease is the presence of uremic symptoms. Uremic symptoms are a collection of clinical symptoms and signs associated with the accumulation of metabolic waste products in the body due to declining kidney function. These symptoms can include nausea, vomiting, fatigue, itching, and mental confusion. They indicate that the kidneys are no longer able to sufficiently remove waste products from the blood, and dialysis is required to perform this function.

(79) (C) Subclavian catheter.

The subclavian approach should be avoided in all patients requiring permanent access later due to the risk of subclavian stenosis.

(80) (B) Buttonhole.

Buttonhole cannulation is associated with an increased infection risk and complications like septic emboli and metastatic seeding. As a result, buttonhole cannulation should only be used in exceptional circumstances like those with short or limited cannulation length and large aneurysmal fistulas.

(81) (B) Arteriovenous fistula (AVF).

The most commonly used type of vascular access for long-term hemodialysis treatments in patients is the arteriovenous fistula (AVF). An atrioventricular fistula is a surgically created connection between an artery and a vein, mostly in the forearm or upper arm (Radial-Basilic AV fistula). Over time, the AVF develops into a more significant, durable, high-flow access site that can accommodate the repeated needle insertions required for hemodialysis.

(82) (B) AVFs have a lower risk of infection than AVGs.

Over time, the AVF develops into a more significant, durable, high-flow access site that can accommodate the repeated needle insertions required for hemodialysis. AVFs are preferred for long-term hemodialysis because they are durable, have high blood flow, and have a lower risk of infection and clotting. AVFs may take several weeks to months for the fistula to mature and become suitable for dialysis.

(83) (C) Hypocalcemia.

“Hypocalcemia” is an electrolyte imbalance that is more likely to occur during hemodialysis and may require supplementation during treatment. Calcium, other waste products, and excess fluids can be removed from the blood during hemodialysis.

Additionally, administration of citrate-containing dialysate solutions can also chelate calcium ions and further contributes to hypocalcemia.

(84) (C) In the dialyzer.

Ultrafiltration occurs within the dialyzer during the hemodialysis process. The dialyzer is a component of the hemodialysis machine; it consists of a semi-permeable membrane that separates the patient's blood from the dialysate solution. As blood and the dialysate flow through the dialyzer, waste products, excess fluid, and electrolytes are exchanged through diffusion across the semi-permeable membrane. Ultrafiltration refers explicitly to removal of excess fluid from the patient's bloodstream through this semi-permeable membrane.

(85) (A) Concentration gradients.

Concentration gradients drive the diffusion of solutes across the dialyzer membrane. Small solutes move from areas of higher concentration (in the patient's blood) to areas of lower concentration (in the dialysate) through diffusion.

(86) (B) Creatinine.

Creatinine is cleared less efficiently in hemodialysis due to its larger size than smaller molecules like urea. Larger molecules have slower transfer rates through the dialyzer membrane.

(87) (C) Control of fluid balance.

The primary objective of ultrafiltration is to regulate fluid equilibrium through elimination of surplus fluid from the patient's circulatory system. This process aids in prevention of conditions such as fluid overload and hypertension.

(88) (C) Hollow-fiber dialyzers

Hollow-fiber dialyzers allow for precise ultrafiltration control and are well-suited for reuse. They maintain a low blood volume relative to their surface area, which enables precise ultrafiltration control.

(89) (B) Ability to handle a high volume of blood.

Hollow-fiber dialyzers are used in modern hemodialysis and are characterized by their ability to handle a high volume of blood, which distinguishes them from parallel plate dialyzers. These dialyzers contain thousands of tiny hollow fibers, through which blood flows, while dialysate flows around these fibers. The design of hollow-fiber dialyzers allows for efficient blood flow and maximizes contact between the blood and the dialysate, which increases the efficiency of waste removal and fluid balance.

(90) (C) Hollow-fiber dialyzers.

Hollow-fiber dialyzers are commonly used in contemporary practice in the USA. They offer advantages like precise ultrafiltration control and minimal resistance to blood flow.

(91) (B) Hollow fiber.

Hollow fiber dialyzers consist of bundles of capillary tubes with polyurethanes, which makes them highly biocompatible. Hollow fiber dialyzers are highly efficient and require low blood primer volume. Above all, they are readily available.

(92) (B) When the toxic substance is known to be dialyzable.

Dialysis is a critical treatment option in cases of acute poisoning, especially when the toxic substance is known to be dialyzable. Dialysis can effectively remove certain toxins from the bloodstream, and significantly help to treat poisoning.

(93) (A) Blood pressure, pulse, temperature, flow rate, and respiratory rate.

These are the parameters that are commonly monitored before and during dialysis as they can indicate how well the patient is tolerating the procedure.

(94) (B) It utilizes reverse osmosis.

In reverse osmosis, solutes move high concentrations to low concentrations across a semipermeable membrane. As the dialysate and blood flow through the dialyzer in opposite directions, a pressure develops that pulls wastes out of the blood into the dialysate.

(95) (C) Magnesium, sodium, and potassium

Dialysate is the fluid used in dialysis, and usually contains a combination of electrolytes such as magnesium, sodium, and potassium. These electrolytes facilitate the diffusion of substances between the blood and the dialysate. Iron and carbon are not usually components of dialysate solutions.

(96) (B) Muscle cramps.

Muscle cramps are a common complication for dialysis patients that can be associated with inappropriate sodium levels in the dialysate. When the sodium concentration in the dialysate is not properly balanced with the patient's serum sodium level, it can cause fluid and electrolyte imbalances.

(97) (B) Low sodium concentration in the dialysate.

Chronic low blood pressure during hemodialysis sessions can be related to a low sodium concentration in the dialysate. A lower concentration of sodium in the dialysate compared to the patient's blood can cause a decrease in osmotic pressure. This reduction can cause fluid to move from the blood into the interstitial spaces, resulting in lower blood pressure.

(98) (B) Sodium.

Persistent fatigue and weakness can be symptoms of dialysis disequilibrium syndrome, which can occur if the sodium content of the dialysate is not correctly adjusted to the patient's serum sodium levels. The rapid removal of urea during dialysis can cause cerebral edema if the serum sodium is not properly balanced. Reviewing and adjusting the sodium content in the dialysate might help to alleviate these symptoms.

(99) (A) Bicarbonate.

Bicarbonate in the blood combines with excess hydrogen ions to form carbonic acid. This compound is then converted into water and carbon dioxide by the enzyme carbonic anhydrase, a process that helps to neutralize metabolic acidosis.

(100) (D) Potassium.

Removing excess potassium from the patient's blood during hemodialysis will correct the hyperkalemia. This can be achieved by adjusting the potassium concentration in the dialysate.

(101) (A) Low blood pressure readings above 150 mmHg.

A blood pressure of 150 mmHg is regarded as hypertension.

(102) (D) All of the above.

The general measures for managing hypotension include decreasing dialysate temperature, putting the patient in Trendelenburg position, and infusing 0.9% saline or 20% albumin.

(103) (B) Decrease in systolic blood pressure by >20–30 mmHg from pre-dialysis levels.

Hypotension is defined by low blood pressure. It is also indicated by either decreased systolic blood pressure by about >20–30 mmHg from pre-dialysis pressure or systolic blood pressure of <100 mmHg.

(104) (A) Hypernatremia.

Some predisposing factors of hypotension include large plasma volume removal, thermal energy transfer that causes vasodilatation, autonomic dysfunction, antihypertensive medications, underlying heart diseases, dehydration, and electrolyte derangements such as hyponatremia.

(105) (B) Dialysis disequilibrium syndrome.

Dialysis disequilibrium syndrome is a set of neurologic and systemic symptoms of varying severity that occur primarily due to cerebral edema in dialyzed patients.

(106) (D) All except (B).

Muscle cramps can be caused by intravascular volume depletion, rapid sodium removal, hyponatremia, and hypotension.

(107) (A) Hypochloremia.

The most common of these electrolyte disturbances are hypo/hyperkalemia, hypo/hypercalcemia, hypo/hypernatremia, and hypomagnesemia.

(108) (C) Both A and B.

The cause of cerebral edema in dialysis disequilibrium syndrome has been proposed by two theories: a reversal of osmotic shift induced by urea removal and a fall in intracellular pH.

(109) (B) Terminate the procedure.

The appropriate thing to do is to terminate the hemodialysis procedure, identify the cause, and treat it.

(110) (A) They are self-limiting.

Symptoms of dialysis disequilibrium syndrome are generally self-limiting and usually resolve within hours.

(111) (A) Poor physical fitness and stamina.

The most likely psychosocial aspect responsible for the patient's frequent job changes is poor physical fitness and stamina. Hemodialysis patients experience fatigue and reduced stamina, which can significantly impact their ability to maintain regular employment.

(112) (C) Difficulty adapting to a new dialysis modality.

The transition from peritoneal dialysis to hemodialysis can be psychologically daunting, as patients face difficulties adapting to a new dialysis modality. Other fears may be present and require some educational efforts from the healthcare provider (e.g., physician, nurse).

(113) (C) Screen measures for anxiety and depression.

Assessing the mental health of hemodialysis patients involves screening measures, such as the Beck Depression Inventory and Hospital Anxiety and Depression Scale. The first option suggests pre-therapeutic counseling, which is both unnecessary and resource intensive. Remember that hemodialysis patients require psychological support (i.e., talk therapy) and not psychiatric intervention. The latter is reserved for severe cases with symptoms that meet the diagnostic criteria of mood disorders (e.g., major depressive disorder).

(114) (B) Selective serotonin reuptake inhibitors (SSRIs).

The main pharmacological treatment for depression in hemodialysis patients includes selective serotonin reuptake inhibitors (SSRIs), such as fluoxetine and sertraline. Close monitoring is recommended due to the risk of bleeding associated with SSRIs. Other antidepressants may be used if patients do not respond to SSRIs or demonstrate refractory depression.

(115) (B) Staphylococcus aureus.

In this clinical scenario, the patient presents with symptoms of a localized infection at the dialysis catheter site. Staphylococcus aureus is a common pathogen responsible for catheter-related infections in hemodialysis patients. Streptococcus pyogenes may also cause skin infections, such as cellulitis, erysipelas, and scarlet fever. However, Staph aureus is more common.

(116) (C) Wash hands frequently.

Washing hands frequently is an important action for nurses to lower the risk of microbial transmission during aseptic procedures in a hemodialysis unit. Hand hygiene is one of the most effective measures to prevent the spread of infections in healthcare settings.

(117) (A) Dispose of it directly after the session.

The nurse should dispose of the ampoule labeled for single use directly after the session. Its reuse would compromise its sterility and is not recommended for infection control. The third option suggests preserving resources. However, this goes against all recognized guidelines.

(118) (C) Proper disinfection of dialysis stations between patients.

Proper disinfection of dialysis stations between patients is vital to lower the risk of blood contamination. This includes cleaning surfaces and containers frequently touched by patients. Although the second option states that surfaces should be cleaned, the method is not sufficient. A clean cloth and water cannot possibly eradicate all the microbes transmitted by patients.

(119) (B) A 1:10 dilution of household bleach.

A 1:10 dilution of household bleach is an effective disinfectant for cleaning areas contaminated with blood in a hemodialysis unit. This concentration is sufficient to kill pathogens, including bloodborne viruses, while being safe for use on most surfaces.

(120) (B) Gowns.

Healthcare staff should wear gowns as part of their personal protective equipment when they perform procedures with a risk of blood spatter during hemodialysis. Gowns protect both staff and patients from potential contamination. Surgical masks are also indispensable. However, masks are almost always worn regardless of the procedure, whereas gowns may be neglected.

(121) (B) Diabetes.

In patients with CKD, diabetes is a common underlying condition that can contribute to a lack of response to recombinant human erythropoietin treatment for anemia. Diabetes can cause conditions such as chronic inflammation and reduced renal function, which can interfere with the body's response to erythropoietin.

(122) (A) It decreases ergosterol synthesis by interfering with cytochrome P450 activity, which inhibits cell membrane formation.

Fluconazole is an antifungal agent which interferes with cytochrome P450 activity and decreases ergosterol synthesis.

(123) (B) It induces erythropoiesis.

In dialysis patients with end-stage renal disease, headache is a common problem. It is often treated with recombinant human erythropoietin. It induces erythropoiesis and binds to its receptor, which is JAK-STAT kinase binding receptor.

(124) (A) It is a polymer of two sulfated disaccharide units: D-glucosamine-L-iduronic acid and D-glucosamine-D-glucuronic acid.

Heparin is a common anticoagulant for dialysis patients. It is a nonuniform mixture of mucopolysaccharides. The molecular weight of heparin is between 10,000 and 20,000. It contains polymers of D-glucosamine-L-iduronic acid and D-glucosamine-D-glucuronic acid.

(125) (C) Only thirty percent of the daily dose is to be used.

The modified dosing of gentamicin in cases of renal insufficiency is summarized below:

- Give seventy percent of the daily recommended dose if creatinine clearance is 70 ml/min.
- Give fifty percent of the daily recommended dose if creatinine clearance is 50 ml/min.
- Give thirty percent of the daily recommended dose if clearance is 30 ml/min.
- Give sixty percent of the daily recommended dose if creatinine clearance is 10-30 ml/min.
- Give forty percent of the daily recommended dose if creatinine clearance is <10 ml/min.

(126) (B) It acts indirectly by activating plasma antithrombin III.

Heparin exerts its anticoagulation property indirectly, as it is responsible for activating antithrombin. A heparin-antithrombin complex forms when heparin binds to antithrombin. This complex binds to clotting factors involved in various coagulation activation pathways. Some common clotting factors heparin inhibits are Xa, IXa, XIIa, and XIIIa. This makes heparin an effective anticoagulant agent both in vitro and in vivo. Heparin does not activate factor VIIa. It is a factor involved in the extrinsic pathway of coagulation. Heparin administered at low doses can affect the conversion of prothrombin to thrombin.

(127) (B) Intravenous administration of salbutamol.

In patients with life-threatening hyperkalemia, administration of intravenous salbutamol can be effective. Dialysis patients are advised to have strict dietary control and completely avoid potassium-rich foods to prevent hyperkalemia. Bicarbonate can be used to correct the potassium level in this patient, but it is not reliable to control potassium levels.

(128) (A) Calcium-containing phosphate binders.

Phosphate binders are the first line of treatment to manage hyperphosphatemia in patients with end-stage renal disease. Aluminum-containing phosphate binders can also prevent and manage hyperphosphatemia in these patients. However, they can cause aluminum toxicity and result in harmful side effects like myopathy, encephalopathy, and failure to treat with erythropoietin.

(129) (A) Kidneys convert Vitamin D to its active form, which is affected in chronic kidney conditions.

In patients with end-stage renal disease undergoing dialysis, vitamin D is significantly reduced due to physiological disturbance in the kidney. These patients are treated with calcitriol, which is the active form of vitamin D.

(130) (B) Hyperparathyroidism.

Cinacalcet is a commonly used drug to manage secondary hyperparathyroidism in dialysis patients. Cinacalcet decreases the level of parathyroid hormone.

(131) (B) Anti-HBV vaccine.

The level of HBsAb should be measured 6 to 12 weeks after patients finish the vaccination series.

(132) (C) Hypokalemia.

In the European phase II trials, sirolimus was associated with hypokalemia compared to cyclosporine.

(133) (B) Hyperchloremia.

Hyperchloremia is not usually a side effect of cyclosporine. Cyclosporine is an immunosuppressive medication that is used in transplant patients. It is known for a variety of side effects, but altering chloride levels is not commonly among them. Common side effects of cyclosporine include hypertension (high blood pressure), gingival hyperplasia (gum enlargement), and hirsutism (excessive hair growth).

(134) (D) Interventional radiology consultation.

For a patient with absent flow in the renal vein post-transplant, as indicated by Doppler ultrasound, the best next step is to consult interventional radiology. This approach aims to assess the situation more thoroughly and determine the most appropriate intervention, which may include procedures to restore blood flow or other therapeutic measures.

(135) (D) Ureteral stent.

If a post-transplant patient shows absent urine output despite a full urinary bladder, inserting a ureteral stent is appropriate. This intervention can help alleviate any obstruction in the urinary tract, which could be responsible for the lack of urine output.

(136) (A) Focal segmental glomerular sclerosis.

FSGS is associated with a 30% recurrence rate after the first and 80% after the subsequent transplantation. The risk of recurrence is higher in patients with familial FSGS, in those with rapid progression to CKD, and at a younger age at transplantation.

(137) (B) Sputum gene X-pert.

The patient presented with symptoms that are suggestive of tuberculosis. The chest x-ray also supports the diagnosis. However, anti-TB treatment should be started once the diagnosis is confirmed. Sputum gene X-pert is the ideal investigative modality to confirm TB.

(138) (C) Rifabutin.

Rifabutin is a drug in the rifamycin family with a lower potential for drug interaction because of its reduced ability to induce cytochrome P450 CYP 3 A and CYP 2 C enzymes.

(139) (A) Bronchoalveolar lavage.

The immunosuppressive medications predispose kidney transplant patients to opportunistic infections, one of which is pneumocystis jirovecii (PCP) pneumonia. The patient's clinical presentation and imaging findings are consistent with this infection. Also, as was seen in this patient, a respiratory system examination could be normal in patients with PCP pneumonia. Induced sputum has a 50-90% sensitivity, whereas bronchoalveolar lavage has a diagnostic yield of more than 90%.

(140) (B) SpO2 less than 88%.

In the described patient with respiratory symptoms, an SpO2 (oxygen saturation) level of less than 88% warrants the use of corticosteroids. This low SpO2 indicates significant oxygenation impairment, which corticosteroids can help improve by reducing inflammation.

(141) (C) Place them in designated bags.

The recommended action to ensure infection control with disposable items that get contaminated with blood is to place them in designated bags that prevent leakage. Proper disposal of contaminated items is vital to protect the facility from contamination. The other options are not effective in isolating the microbes.

(142) (B) A confirmed infection.

A confirmed infection is the only factor that justifies the isolation of the patient. Vague symptoms of inflammation are not indicative of any diagnosis and further investigation should be conducted. Her history of diabetes may put her at risk of immunosuppression, which increases the risk of some infections. However, this is not an indication of isolation. The patient also reports that she did not receive the hepatitis B vaccine. This option is a distractor despite the importance of this vaccine in this subset of patients.

(143) (B) Maintain catheter sterility.

The purpose of examining the catheter exit site is to look for signs of infection and maintain catheter sterility. The other options are relatively correct. However, they do not justify the regular examination of the catheter exit site.

(144) (D) Osteoporosis as its risk increases due to long-term heparin use.

Long-term heparin use, especially in high doses, increases the risk of osteoporosis. Colle's fracture and bone pain suggest osteoporosis secondary to heparin therapy, as the patient has been taking heparin and undergoing dialysis for more than three years. Heparin has no relation with osteosarcoma, osteoarthritis, or osteophyte formation.

(145) (B) Cinacalcet.

Cinacalcet manages secondary hyperparathyroidism. It decreases the parathyroid hormone level by activating the calcium-sensing receptor, which is normally in the parathyroid gland.

(146) (B) Varicella vaccine.

Since it is a live vaccine, the varicella vaccine is contraindicated in kidney transplant patients. Thus, it should be administered 4-6 weeks prior to transplantation.

(147) (C) It should be given because the rabies vaccine is safe for immunosuppressed patients.

The rabies vaccine is an inactivated vaccine. It is safe for renal transplant patients. Hence, they should receive the vaccine per recommendation for the general population.

(148) (D) No additional intervention is required.

This patient has a slowly recovering graft function. These patients do not require support with dialysis unless they have an electrolyte abnormality, fluid overload, or severe anemia requiring a blood transfusion.

(149) (B) Urine culture.

A urine culture should be obtained before empirical therapy is started. Then, after the culture and sensitivity results are available, definitive treatment is started.

(150) (B) New onset proteinuria.

KIDGO suggests a renal biopsy for patients with new-onset proteinuria. The rest of the choices in the question are not indications for biopsy.

Test 3 Questions

(1) Which of the following is not a microstructure of the kidney?

(A) Renal fascia.

(B) Proximal convoluted tubule.

(C) Loop of Henle.

(D) Collecting ducts.

(2) Which of the following is a feature of the renal corpuscle?

(A) It is formed by the proximal convoluted tubule and the renal fascia.

(B) The renal corpuscle is responsible for the filtration of blood.

(C) Blood enters the glomerulus through the efferent arteriole.

(D) Blood leaves the glomerulus through the afferent arteriole.

(3) Which of the following is true about the proximal convoluted tubule?

(A) It is the coiled initial portion of the nephron that arises from loop of Henle.

(B) It continues as the collecting duct.

(C) It is formed by 3 layers of flat epithelium that interdigitate.

(D) The primary role of the proximal convoluted tubule is the reabsorption of water and electrolytes.

(4) Which is not a part of the loop of Henle?

(A) The descending limb.

(B) Hairpin bend.

(C) Thick distal convoluted tubule.

(D) The ascending limb.

(5) Which of the following is true about the distal convoluted tubule?

(A) The distal convoluted tubule is about 14–15 cm in length.

(B) It is lined by a layer of cuboidal epithelium called intercalated cells.

(C) It continues as the proximal convoluted tubule.

(D) The thick descending segment of the loop of Henle continues as the distal convoluted tubule.

(6) Which of the following structures does not form the juxtaglomerular apparatus?

(A) Macula densa.

(B) Mesangial cells.

(C) Juxtaglomerular cells.

(D) Renin cells.

(7) Which of the following is not true about juxtaglomerular cells?

(A) They form part of the juxtaglomerular apparatus.

(B) They are smooth muscle cells containing secretory granules within their cytoplasm.

(C) They are present in the tunica media and the tunica adventitia of the afferent arteriole.

(D) They are a condensation of cells of the terminal portion of the collecting duct.

(8) Which of the following is one of the functions of the juxtaglomerular apparatus?

(A) The juxtaglomerular apparatus secretes hormones, which include renin and prostaglandins.

(B) It regulates erythropoiesis.

(C) It plays a role in the synthesis of vitamin D.

(D) It plays a role in the synthesis of thrombopoietin.

(9) Which of the following is not true about the formation of angiotensin II?

(A) Renin catalyzes the conversion of angiotensinogen to angiotensin I, which is physiologically inactive.

(B) The cascade of reactions is stimulated by a fall in arterial blood pressure, reduced extracellular fluid volume, and reduced sodium chloride concentration.

(C) Angiotensin I is converted to angiotensin II by an angiotensin-converting enzyme produced in the lungs.

(D) Angiotensin is converted to angiotensin I.

(10) Which of the following is true about the action of angiotensin II?

(A) It is a potent venous vasoconstrictor that increases blood pressure by vasodilation.

(B) It also decreases the release of noradrenaline from postganglionic sympathetic fibers.

(C) It causes constriction of the efferent arteriole, which results in decreased glomerular filtration rate.

(D) It stimulates the baroreceptor reflex.

(11) A 28-year-old female patient presents with a history of systemic lupus erythematosus. She complains of proteinuria and swelling in her ankles. What type of kidney disease is commonly associated with systemic lupus erythematosus?

(A) IgG4-related disease.

(B) Membranous nephropathy.

(C) Hemophagocytic condition.

(D) Henoch Schönlein purpura.

(12) A 10-year-old child is brought to the pediatric clinic by their parents. The parents are concerned about a sudden onset of abdominal pain. Upon examination, the child is found to have small red and purple dots on their lower extremities, as well as joint pain and abdominal tenderness. The child does not have a history of trauma or known allergies. There is no significant family history of similar symptoms. Based on the clinical presentation, what vessels are most likely targeted in this condition?

(A) Arteries.

(B) Veins.

(C) Small blood vessels.

(D) Lymphatic vessels.

(13) A 45-year-old patient presents with vasculitis-mediated kidney disease. Laboratory tests reveal IgA autoantibodies. What is the most likely diagnosis?

(A) Hemophagocytic disease.

(B) IgG4-related disease.

(C) Henoch Schönlein purpura.

(D) Systemic lupus erythematosus.

(14) What is the mnemonic used to remember the key clinical features of Henoch Schönlein purpura, which causes kidney disease?

(A) PAAN.

(B) HEMO.

(C) RENA.

(D) IGAA.

(15) Which target organ is not commonly affected by heavy metal exposure?

(A) Central nervous system.

(B) Liver.

(C) Lungs.

(D) Skin.

(16) In chronic exposure to heavy metals, what form of heavy metals is generally conjugated by glutathione and metallothionein?

(A) Protein-bound form.

(B) Ionized form.

(C) Gaseous form.

(D) Solid form.

(17) During acute heavy metal toxicity, which parts of the kidney are involved in the reabsorption of ionized metals?

(A) Proximal tubule and loop of Henle.

(B) Distal tubule and collecting duct.

(C) Glomerulus and Bowman's capsule.

(D) Ureter and bladder.

(18) What should clinicians consider when a patient's kidney disease cannot be attributed to common etiologies?

(A) Shift focus to the patient's lifestyle.

(B) Order more imaging tests.

(C) Explore the family history of renal disease.

(D) Prescribe furosemide to control symptoms.

(19) Research has shown that a single-gene defect may be responsible for certain kidney diseases. What is an example of a gene mutation that causes kidney disease?

(A) Dystrophin gene.

(B) Podocin gene.

(C) CFTR gene.

(D) HEXA gene.

(20) What potential treatment for genetic renal disease is being researched?

(A) Use of targeted drugs.

(B) Increased reliance on surgical interventions.

(C) Focus on lifestyle modifications.

(D) Exploration of alternative medicine.

(21) Which of the following best defines how stage 1 chronic kidney disease is usually diagnosed?

(A) By urine color.

(B) By the presence of physical symptoms.

(C) By assessment of albuminuria or other signs of kidney damage.

(D) By blood pressure measurement.

(22) Which of the following is the primary goal of management of stage 1 CKD?

(A) To prevent further kidney damage.

(B) To provide immediate dialysis.

(C) To reverse the damage already done.

(D) To improve kidney function.

(23) A 45-year-old known diabetic man has an eGFR of 40 mL/min/1.73m^2 and moderate proteinuria. He also complained of fatigue and swelling in the ankles. Which of the following is not likely to be true concerning this patient?

(A) He is in stage 3 CKD.

(B) He is likely to have hyperphosphatemia.

(C) His ankle edema likely resulted from right-sided heart failure.

(D) His management plan should aim to slow disease progression, manage symptoms, and address complications.

(24) Albumin excretion values in the range of 30-300 mg/24hr indicate which of the following stages of CKD?

(A) Stage 1.

(B) Stage 2.

(C) Stage 3.

(D) Stage 4.

(25) CKD can be classified based on which of the following?

(1) eGFR category (G1-G5).

(2) Albuminuria category (A1-A3).

(3) Age.

(4) Ethnicity.

(A) 1 and 4.

(B) 1 only.

(C) 1 and 2.

(D) All of the above.

(26) The definition of CKD is based on the following criteria:

(1) eGFR less than 60 mL/min/1.73m^2

(2) Albuminuria (urine albumin excretion rate greater than or equal to 30 mg/24hr; urine albumin-creatinine ratio (greater than or equal to 3 mg/mmol).

(3) Urine sediment abnormalities.

(4) Renal tubular disorders.

(5) Pathological and structural abnormalities.

These criteria should be present for how many months to diagnose CKD?

(A) One month.

(B) Two months.

(C) Three months.

(D) Four months.

(27) In the evaluation of a 55-year-old man for dialysis, he was noticed to be receiving Epoetin alfa three times per week. The patient's current lab results are;

- Hemoglobin: 8 g/dL.
- Ferritin: 300 μ/L.
- Transferrin saturation: 25%.
- Vitamin B12: Within normal levels.
- Folate: Within normal levels.

What course of treatment would you recommend for this patient?

(A) Increase the Epoetin alfa dosage.

(B) Decrease the Epoetin alfa dosage.

(C) No change in the Epoetin alfa dosage.

(D) Discontinue the Epoetin alfa therapy.

(28) Which of the following is the likely mechanism responsible for increased susceptibility to infection in patients with chronic kidney disease?

(A) Increase renal deposition of sugar and solutes.

(B) Urinary loss of antithrombin III.

(C) Urinary loss of complement proteins.

(D) Accumulation of fluid in the interstitial compartment.

(29) In staging chronic kidney disease using the eGFR, what is the eGFR range for stage 4 CKD?

(A) 45-59 mL/min/1.73m^2.

(B) 30-44 mL/min/1.73m^2.

(C) 15-29 mL/min/1.73m^2.

(D) Less than 15 mL/min/1.73m^2.

(30) Which stage of CKD is characterized by kidney damage with a normal eGFR value?

(A) None.

(B) Stage 1.

(C) Stage 2.

(D) Stage 3.

(31) Which of the following is not a common complication of CKD?

(A) Hyperkalemia.

(B) Metabolic alkalosis.

(C) Osteoporosis.

(D) Anemia.

(32) Which of the following conditions is a common cause of postrenal AKI?

(A) Acute tubular necrosis.

(B) Glomerulonephritis.

(C) Benign prostatic hyperplasia.

(D) Acute interstitial nephritis.

(33) Which of the following medications should be avoided in patients with AKI due to its potential nephrotoxic effects?

(A) Amoxicillin.

(B) Acetaminophen.

(C) Ibuprofen.

(D) Diphenhydramine.

(34) Which of these is the treatment of choice for patients with ESKD when GFR falls to 5–10 mL/min/1.73m^2?

(A) Hemodialysis.

(B) Peritoneal dialysis.

(C) Kidney transplantation.

(D) Palliative care.

(35) Which factor significantly influences the prognosis of CKD?

(A) The stage of CKD.

(B) The patient's age.

(C) A sudden onset of symptoms.

(D) The reversible nature of the condition.

(36) What is the main objective of renal replacement therapy in ESKD?

(A) To cure patients with CKD.

(B) To slow down disease progression in patients with CKD.

(C) To improve the quality of life and long-term survival in patients with CKD.

(D) To reverse kidney damage in patients with CKD.

(37) What is the primary objective in the management of patients with AKI?

(A) To cure AKI.

(B) To reverse kidney damage.

(C) To slow down CKD progression.

(D) To prevent further deterioration and restore function.

(38) What is the main indication for kidney transplants in patients with End-Stage Kidney Disease?

(A) Hypertension that is difficult to control.

(B) Significant decline in the glomerular filtration rate.

(C) Development of secondary hyperparathyroidism.

(D) Presence of diabetic nephropathy.

(39) Which of the following is a common cause of prerenal AKI?

(A) Acute glomerulonephritis.

(B) Renal artery thrombosis.

(C) Tubular necrosis.

(D) Nephrotoxic medications.

(40) What is the primary goal of dietary management for patients with CKD?

(A) Limit fluid intake.

(B) Control protein intake.

(C) Restrict carbohydrate intake.

(D) Increase potassium-rich foods.

(41) Excess magnesium in the blood can also elevate blood levels in circulation due to kidney disease. Which of the following terms defines this occurrence?

(A) Hyponatremia.

(B) Hypermagnesemia.

(C) Hypomagnesemia.

(D) Hyperphosphatemia.

(42) Which of the following symptoms could people with chronic kidney disease and acid-base imbalances display as a result of respiratory compensation?

(A) Increased blood pressure.

(B) Rapid breathing.

(C) Slurred speech.

(D) Decreased heart rate.

(43) Mrs. Johnson has had chronic disease for some time and her blood work results demonstrate elevated potassium levels. What appropriate dietary modification is fit for her?

(A) Potassium restriction.

(B) Protein restriction.

(C) Sodium restriction.

(D) Intake of breads and cereals.

(44) A nurse from the last shift notes that Andrew sustained a fracture due to altered calcium and phosphorus metabolism. What process might have cause this?

(A) Aluminum loss through the impaired kidney functions.

(B) Calcium and phosphate deposition in tissues.

(C) Decreased absorption of calcium due to impaired vitamin D activation.

(D) Parathyroid hormone increases because of low calcium levels.

(45) During your regular duty as a nurse you review Max's blood results. He is a 70-year-old man with chronic kidney disease and his potassium levels are off the chart. Which food type would you advise against?

(A) Consumption of cheese and yogurt.

(B) Consumption of spinach and kale.

(C) Consumption of white bread and pasta.

(D) Consumption of bananas and oranges.

(46) Which of the following statements below is accurate about secondary hypertension in patients with chronic kidney disease?

(A) Hypertension is not a risk factor for increased cardiovascular complications in patients with chronic kidney disease.

(B) Hypertension causes a progressive fall in kidney function in chronic kidney disease patients.

(C) Hypertension cannot lead to heart failure in chronic kidney disease.

(D) It's very easy to regulate blood pressure in patients with chronic kidney disease.

(47) In patients with CKD, what is a common symptom associated with hypernatremia, or excess sodium in the body?

(A) Decreased urine output.

(B) Swelling in the feet and legs.

(C) Severe headaches.

(D) Sudden weight loss.

(48) Which of the following statements is accurate about anemia in chronic kidney disease?

(A) Anemia is found in 50% of patients with advanced chronic kidney disease.

(B) Anemia in chronic kidney disease has no effects on quality of life.

(C) Patients with CKD frequently experience absolute iron deficiency, but functional iron deficiency is rare.

(D) Iron deficiency in normal kidney patients is constant and similar to patients with chronic kidney disease.

(49) Mineral and bone disorders in patients with chronic kidney disease can be accurately described by which statement below?

(A) Skeletal complications are rare in chronic kidney disease patients.

(B) Vitamin D supplementation is only given to patients with advanced chronic kidney disease.

(C) Mineral and bone disorders present no risk for cardiovascular disease in patients with chronic kidney disease.

(D) Mineral and bone disorders may present risk of premature death in chronic kidney disease patients as well as increased risk for cardiovascular disease and its associated complications.

(50) How frequent should cardiovascular risk be assessed in chronic kidney disease patients due to non-specific signs and symptoms that could result from other organs or derangements?

(A) Every 8 months.

(B) Every 6 months.

(C) Every 9 months.

(D) After every 2 years.

(51) A know chronic kidney disease patient starts feeling confused with muscle cramps and irregularities in the heart beat pattern. Laboratory results show near normal levels of potassium. Which other electrolyte can cause this condition?

(A) Hyperphosphatemia.

(B) Hypercalcemia.

(C) Hypermagnesemia.

(D) Hypocalcemia.

(52) A 55-year-old male patient with chronic kidney disease has elevated blood pressure. He presents with edema of the legs, difficulty breathing, and fatigue. What cardiovascular complication might this represent?

(A) Peripheral arterial disease.

(B) Congestive heart failure.

(C) Coronary artery disease.

(D) Atrial fibrillation.

(53) A 72-year-old male patient with a long history of hypertension and chronic kidney disease presents with palpitations. Later his ECG findings reveal absent p waves. What cardiovascular complication is present?

(A) Hypertensive crisis.

(B) Myocardial infarction.

(C) Hyperkalemia.

(D) Atrial fibrillation.

(54) Renal osteodystrophy, a condition associated with chronic kidney disease, is characterized by which of the following changes?

(A) Increased red blood cell production.

(B) Improved glucose metabolism.

(C) Altered bone metabolism and remodeling.

(D) Enhanced gastrointestinal function.

(55) A 65-year-old man with chronic kidney disease is admitted for chest pain and shortness of breath during physical activity. Left ventricular hypertrophy findings are noted on ECG. Which of the following is the cause of the left ventricular hypertrophy?

(A) Hypocalcemia.

(B) Hyperkalemia.

(C) Anemia.

(D) Hypertension.

(56) A 78-year-old man presents with complaints of chest pains centrally located that get worse whenever he breathes in. This has been ongoing for some time. He attributes worsening symptoms to his kidney failure problem that was diagnosed 20 years ago. On auscultation there is a pericardial friction rub. What might cause the problem in this patient?

(A) Hypercalcemia.

(B) Uremic pericarditis.

(C) Left ventricular hypertrophy.

(D) Anemia.

(57) In which of the following scenarios is an acute anuria (absence of urine) in a young patient least likely to indicate the need for a renal biopsy?

(A) The patient has a history of chronic kidney disease.

(B) The patient is showing signs of systemic lupus erythematosus.

(C) There is no clear underlying risk factor for the anuria.

(D) The patient has recently started new medications known to affect kidney function.

(58) A 35-year-old male patient presents with reddish discoloration of urine, a decrease in urine amount, and hemoptysis. Urine analysis shows RBC in urine and renal function tests indicate increased creatinine. Renal biopsy was done and light microscopy shows crescentic glomerulonephritis. Linear deposition of IgG on glomerular capillaries is also shown in immunofluorescence electron microscopy. Which of the following is the most likely diagnosis of the patient?

(A) Membranous nephropathy.

(B) Lupus nephritis.

(C) Anti-GBM disease.

(D) Focal segmental glomerulosclerosis.

(59) A 40-year-old female patient presents with joint pain, facial rash, easy fatigability, reddish discoloration of urine, and a decrease in the amount of urine. Baseline renal investigations show increased creatinine, positive ANA, and RBC in urine. A renal biopsy is done and an electron microscope shows thickening of the GBM mesangial expansion, endothelial cell swelling, and podocyte foot process effacement. Full house immunofluorescence pattern is also shown. What is the most likely diagnosis?

(A) Membranous nephropathy.

(B) Lupus nephritis.

(C) Anti-GBM disease.

(D) Focal segmental glomerulosclerosis.

(60) Which of the following is not an indication for initiation of dialysis?

(A) Increased creatinine of >10.

(B) Refractory hyperkalemia.

(C) Refractory academia.

(D) Uremic symptoms.

(61) An 18-year-old male patient is on hemodialysis for glomerulonephritis. This results in refractory hyperkalemia. Which of the following complications do you least expect to happen due to the hemodialysis?

(A) Hypotension.

(B) Nonfunctional hemodialysis access.

(C) Anaphylactic reactions to the dialysate.

(D) Peritonitis.

(62) Which of the following is a false statement regarding renal transplantation?

(A) Psychosocial evaluation is an integral part of pre-transplant evaluation to assess the patient's understanding, readiness, and social support.

(B) Deceased donors should be screened for infections and malignancies.

(C) Regular follow-up is key to monitor any complications or signs of rejection.

(D) Induction immunosuppressive therapy is given long-term to prevent rejection.

(63) A 65-year-old woman undergoes a CT scan with contrast for abdominal pain. Two days later, her creatinine increases from 1.0 to 1.8 mg/dL. What is the most appropriate next step?

(A) Start hemodialysis.

(B) Obtain a kidney biopsy.

(C) Stop all nephrotoxic medications.

(D) Reassure the patient this is normal.

(64) Which of the following hormones is not produced by the kidneys?

(A) Erythropoietin.

(B) Angiotensinogen.

(C) Prostaglandins.

(D) Renin.

(65) A 67-year-old male and known hypertensive patient experiences progressively worsening easy fatigability, facial swelling, and decreased amount of urine. His creatinine is 6.8 and there is proteinuria in urine analysis. Which of the following imaging investigations is important to aid with the diagnosis of CKD?

(A) Renal ultrasound.

(B) MRI.

(C) X-ray.

(D) Non-contrast CT.

(66) A 45-year-old woman with lupus undergoes a kidney biopsy. Which vital sign does the nurse monitor every 15 minutes for the first hour after the biopsy?

(A) Respiratory rate.

(B) Blood pressure.

(C) Temperature.

(D) Oxygen saturation.

(67) Which of these types of dialysis is associated with interdialytic fluid accumulation?

(A) Conventional hemodialysis.

(B) Hemofiltration.

(C) Short daily hemodialysis.

(D) Home hemodialysis.

(68) Mr. Y is a 55-year-old ESRD patient on dialysis at home for two to three hours six times a week. Which of these best describes his treatment modality?

(A) Short daily hemodialysis.

(B) In-center nocturnal dialysis.

(C) Short daily home dialysis.

(D) None of the above.

(69) Which of the following is associated with an increased need for antihypertensive medications?

(A) In-center nocturnal dialysis.

(B) Home short daily hemodialysis.

(C) Home nocturnal hemodialysis.

(D) Conventional hemodialysis.

(70) Which of the modalities below uses low-flux dialyzers?

(A) Home nocturnal hemodialysis.

(B) Conventional hemodialysis.

(C) Short daily dialysis.

(D) Hemofiltration.

(71) How does short daily dialysis affect treatment duration and frequency?

(A) The individual sessions are prolonged.

(B) The frequency of sessions is reduced.

(C) Each session is shorter, but they occur more frequently.

(D) Patients undergo dialysis only a few times per week.

(72) Diffusion is the movement of molecules:

(A) Across a pressure gradient.

(B) From a region of high concentration to a region of low concentration.

(C) From a region of low concentration to a region of high concentration.

(D) Via hydrostatic forces.

(73) In-center self-care hemodialysis is done:

(A) At home.

(B) At the center by the nursing staff.

(C) At the center by the patient.

(D) By the care person.

(74) Which of the following is not an advantage of short daily hemodialysis?

(A) Enhanced filtration of toxins.

(B) Improved survival rate.

(C) Heightened risk of vascular access complications.

(D) Improved blood pressure control.

(75) Hemofiltration does not involve the use of any dialysate. In this case, how is the dialysis performed?

(A) Convection only.

(B) Convection and conduction.

(C) Diffusion and convection.

(D) Diffusion only.

(76) A major disadvantage of in-center dialysis compared to home dialysis is:

(A) The inflexible schedule.

(B) The nursing staff administers treatment.

(C) Patients are monitored during the session.

(D) None of the above.

(77) Mrs. Jemila is a 68-year-old woman undergoing hemodialysis treatment for end-stage renal disease through arteriovenous fistula for the past two years. She has recently complained of severe pain and swelling in her left arm during dialysis sessions. She also noticed that her left hand turns pale and cold during dialysis. What is the most likely diagnosis?

(A) Raynaud's phenomenon.

(B) Carpal tunnel syndrome.

(C) Sciatica.

(D) Steal syndrome.

(78) Mr. Keith is a chronic liver disease patient who currently presents with acute decompensation. His serum creatinine is 6.8, and BUN is 120. He is confused and has shortness of breath. Imaging shows pulmonary edema. The managing team decides on emergency hemodialysis. Which route of vascular access is ideal?

(A) Arteriovenous fistula.

(B) Arteriovenous graft.

(C) Central venous catheter.

(D) Intraosseous.

(79) Which two imaging modalities are important in utilizing a central venous catheter during and after insertion?

(A) Ultrasound and x-ray.

(B) X-ray and ultrasound.

(C) Chest CT and MRI.

(D) Ultrasound and CT.

(80) Which one of the following hemodialysis vascular access options carries the highest risk of infection?

(A) AVF.

(B) AVG.

(C) Central venous catheter.

(D) All carry the same risk.

(81) Mr. Hannibal is a CKD patient with AVF on regular hemodialysis. Upon his routine follow-up, his healthcare provider puts a stethoscope on his hand and listens. What is the provider appreciating?

(A) Thrill.

(B) Bruit.

(C) Murmur.

(D) Pulse.

(82) Which of the following is not one of the measures to prevent central venous catheter infection?

(A) Regularly clean catheter exits with iodine or chlorhexidine.

(B) Regularly wash catheter exits with clean water and soap.

(C) Regularly examine for signs of infections.

(D) Regularly dress the catheter exit.

(83) A 35-year-old female patient on hemodialysis for AKI secondary to preeclampsia via a central venous catheter has started to experience fever, chills, and rigor one week after insertion. Blood workup shows leukocytosis of 15,000, with neutrophils comprising 89%. What is the most likely focus of infection?

(A) Chest.

(B) Urinary tract.

(C) Central venous catheter.

(D) GI.

(84) Abel is a new patient who decided to get an AVF for his hemodialysis. He meets you in the hallway and asks, “What should I check for regularly to monitor my AV fistula?” What is the correct answer?

(A) Capillary refill.

(B) Radial pulse.

(C) Thrill or bruit.

(D) Skin temperature.

(85) How can catheter blockages be prevented?

(A) Strict aseptic technique.

(B) Routine catheter replacement.

(C) Adequate flushing and heparin lock.

(D) Area puncture technique.

(86) Which is the most preferred site for arteriovenous fistula?

(A) Brachiocephalic.

(B) Forearm prosthetic graft.

(C) Radiocephalic.

(D) Radiobasilic.

(87) What is the primary material used in modern dialyzer membranes in the United States?

(A) Cellulose.

(B) Polysulfone.

(C) Polyethylene.

(D) Polyvinyl chloride.

(88) What is the standard range for dialysate sodium concentration during hemodialysis?

(A) 120–125 mmol/L.

(B) 136–140 mmol/L.

(C) 145–155 mmol/L.

(D) 0–4 mmol/L

(89) What is the purpose of "sodium modeling" during hemodialysis?

(A) To lower dialysate sodium concentration.

(B) To counterbalance urea-related osmolar gradients.

(C) To increase thirst in patients with hypertension.

(D) To remove excess fluid.

(90) What is the primary purpose of adjustment of the composition of the dialysate solution?

(A) To enhance patient comfort.

(B) To maintain a balanced electrolyte profile.

(C) To reduce the risk of arrhythmias.

(D) To decrease fluid removal.

(91) What treatment is done on the water used for dialysate to eliminate microbiological contaminants and dissolved ions?

(A) Filtration.

(B) Softening.

(C) Deionization.

(D) Reverse osmosis.

(92) What is the most essential vital sign monitored during hemodialysis?

(A) Random blood glucose.

(B) Temperature.

(C) Blood pressure.

(D) Respiratory rate.

(93) Excessive ultrafiltration in hemodialysis may cause:

(A) Raised blood glucose.

(B) Raised temperature.

(C) Dehydration.

(D) Coagulopathy.

(94) Patient monitoring in dialysis is achieved through which of the following?

(A) Vital signs.

(B) Knee jerk reflex.

(C) Abdominal examination.

(D) Muscle bulk.

(95) Why is anticoagulation monitoring necessary during hemodialysis?

(A) To prevent excessive bleeding.

(B) To ensure proper pH levels.

(C) To assess vascular access.

(D) To monitor ultrafiltration rates.

(96) Which of the following helps to prevent potential complications in facilities where dialyzers are reused?

(A) Monitor dialysate composition.

(B) Document patient complaints.

(C) Cleaning and disinfection protocols.

(D) Conduct pre-dialysis assessments.

(97) Through which of the following procedures is vascular access achieved during hemodialysis?

(A) Paul's tubing.

(B) Pulse oximeter.

(C) Laryngoscopy.

(D) Fistula and graft.

(98) What medium helps to filter waste products from blood?

(A) Dialysate.

(B) Fistula and graft.

(C) Alarm system.

(D) Pressure gauge.

(99) Which of these is true concerning the dialyzer in hemodialysis?

(A) Lower blood flow increases efficacy.

(B) Higher blood flow increases efficacy.

(C) Blood flow has no impact.

(D) All of the above.

(100) What is the first step in monitoring the hemodialysis process?

(A) Vascular access assessment.

(B) Hemodynamic monitoring.

(C) Pre-dialysis evaluation.

(D) Dialysate temperature check.

(101) Which dialyzer should be used to efficiently clear beta 2-microglobulin molecules from a sixty-five-year-old hemodialysis patient's blood?

(A) High-flux dialyzer.

(B) Synthetic membrane dialyzer.

(C) Cellulose-based dialyzer.

(D) Low-flux dialyzer.

(102) Why are highly permeable dialyzers (usually made with synthetic membranes) used in hemodialysis?

(A) To increase the speed of the dialysis session.

(B) To minimize biocompatibility-related reactions.

(C) To enhance the removal of large molecules only.

(D) To reduce the need for anticoagulants during dialysis.

(103) What kind of dialyzer is appropriate in a small space?

(A) High-flux dialyzer.

(B) Low-flux dialyzer.

(C) Synthetic membrane dialyzer.

(D) Parallel plate dialyzer.

(104) Which dialyzer type carries the lowest cross-contamination risk?

(A) High-flux dialyzer.

(B) Synthetic membrane dialyzer.

(C) Regenerated cellulose dialyzer.

(D) Hollow fiber dialyzer.

(105) Why are high-flux dialyzers preferred in certain hemodialysis treatments?

(A) They are more cost-effective compared to other types.

(B) They require shorter dialysis sessions.

(C) They effectively remove both small and midsized solutes.

(D) They reduce the need for heparin during dialysis.

(106) Which component of the dialysis machine prevents blood clotting?

(A) Blood pump.

(B) Dialyzer.

(C) Control panel.

(D) An anticoagulant such as heparin.

(107) A fifty-year-old female patient with chronic kidney disease asks how frequently dialysis should be done. What is the appropriate response?

(A) Once per week.

(B) Three times per week.

(C) Every day.

(D) Twice a day.

(108) Which mineral should a dialysis patient consume in cautious moderation?

(A) Potassium.

(B) Iron.

(C) Zinc.

(D) Magnesium.

(109) In hemodialysis, why is potassium carefully controlled and adjusted in the dialysate?

(A) To enhance the patient's calcium absorption.

(B) To prevent blood clotting during dialysis.

(C) To manage the patient's electrolyte balance.

(D) To increase the efficiency of toxin removal.

(110) Which of the below components is not part of dialysate and is not changed in concentration during the hemodialysis session?

(A) The pH.

(B) The urea concentration.

(C) The glucose (dextrose) concentration.

(D) The bicarbonate concentration.

(111) Which of these compounds is added to dialysate to prevent low calcium levels in hemodialysis patients?

(A) Potassium chloride (KCl).

(B) Magnesium sulfate ($MgSO_4$).

(C) Sodium bicarbonate ($NaHCO_3$).

(D) Calcium chloride ($CaCl_2$).

(112) Of the components added to dialysate, which one controls acidosis in hemodialysis patients?

(A) Bicarbonate (HCO_3^-).

(B) Chloride (Cl^-).

(C) Potassium (K^+).

(D) Calcium (Ca^{2+}).

(113) What is the main reason for adding glucose (dextrose) to dialysate for hemodialysis patients?

(A) To raise the pH of the dialysate.

(B) To provide a source of energy for the patient.

(C) To prevent clotting in the dialysis machine.

(D) To control the patient's electrolyte balance.

(114) What is the main rationale for reusing dialyzers?

(A) To reduce costs.

(B) To improve patient comfort.

(C) To maintain the dialyzer's performance.

(D) To reduce the risk of contamination.

(115) How are dialyzers prepared if they are to be reused?

(A) They are stored as is until the next session.

(B) They are subjected to a thorough cleaning and disinfection process.

(C) They are rinsed with water.

(D) They are discarded after a single use.

(116) A patient complains of chest pain while on hemodialysis. Which of the following is not a probable cause?

(A) Angina.

(B) Muscle cramps.

(C) Myocardial infarction.

(D) Air embolism.

(117) Which of the following is true about air embolism?

(A) It is the presence of air in the lungs.

(B) It is not potentially lethal.

(C) It is air trapped in the lungs.

(D) It is the presence of air in the lungs and systemic circulation.

(118) Which of the following is a clinical feature of air embolism?

(A) A pink foamy air pocket in the extracorporeal system venous line.

(B) Cough and shortness of breath.

(C) Chest pain or pressure.

(D) All of the above.

(119) Which of the following steps cannot prevent air embolism?

(A) Keep the level of drip chambers up.

(B) Replace empty saline bags immediately.

(C) Loosen connections when priming.

(D) None of the above.

(120) Which of the following symptoms is often associated with hypocalcemia?

(A) Muscle cramps and twitching.

(B) Extreme thirst.

(C) Confusion and lethargy.

(D) Nausea and vomiting.

(121) Which of the following is the primary mechanism that causes hypotension during hemodialysis?

(A) Excess removal of fluid.

(B) High blood pressure.

(C) Electrolyte imbalances.

(D) Inadequate dialysis time.

(122) Which of the following is anticoagulation is a treatment modality for?

(A) Air embolism.

(B) Clotting.

(C) Dialysis reaction.

(D) Hypotension.

(123) What is the mechanism of hyperkalemia in hemolysis?

(A) Osmosis.

(B) Diffusion.

(C) Release of intracellular potassium.

(D) Release of calcium.

(124) Which of the following mechanisms result in hemolysis?

(A) Excessive negative pressure in the extracorporeal circuit.

(B) Deformity in lines (kinks and folds).

(C) Overocclusion of blood pump.

(D) All of the above.

(125) Which of the following symptoms is not typically associated with dialysis disequilibrium syndrome?

(A) Headache.

(B) Nausea.

(C) Chest pain.

(D) Restlessness.

(126) What is a common cause of itching in dialyzed patients?

(A) Allergic reaction to the dialyzer membrane.

(B) Elevated levels of parathyroid hormone due to primary hyperparathyroidism.

(C) Dehydration during dialysis sessions.

(D) Accumulation of urea in the blood.

(127) Which of the following poses a risk for the development of hypotension during hemodialysis?

(A) Hypertension.

(B) Use of short-acting antihypertensives within 4 hours of dialysis.

(C) Hypernatremia.

(D) Antimicrobials.

(128) Which of the following is a cause of extreme blood loss?

(A) Blood line separation.

(B) Rupture of anastomosis or aneurysm.

(C) Crack in dialyzer casing or rupture of dialyzer.

(D) All of the above.

(129) Which of the following is a dialyzer reaction?

(A) First-use syndrome.

(B) Hypersensitivity to membrane.

(C) Urticaria.

(D) Both A and B.

(130) Which of the following describes first-use syndrome?

(A) It is a severe IgE anaphylactoid reaction.

(B) It usually occurs during the first use of a dialyzer.

(C) Its effects are reproducible during subsequent hemodialysis sessions.

(D) All of the above.

(131) Which of the following has clinical features such as hives, angioedema, urticaria, and pruritus?

(A) Electrolyte derangement.

(B) Muscle cramps.

(C) Dialyzer reactions.

(D) Arrhythmias.

(132) Which is related to hypertension during hemodialysis?

(A) Fluid overload.

(B) Non-compliance with blood pressure medications.

(C) Both A and B.

(D) None of the above.

(133) Which of the following can help you manage a dialyzer reaction?

(A) Antihypertensive.

(B) Antibiotics.

(C) Treatment with epinephrine and steroids.

(D) Anticoagulation.

(134) Which of the following can help you manage itching?

(A) Adequate dialysis to regulate electrolyte levels.

(B) Lotions or medications for dry skin or allergies.

(C) Control of uremia and secondary hyperparathyroidism.

(D) All of the above.

(135) Which of the following describes a reaction due to presence of dead bacteria and/or endotoxins within the systemic circulation?

(A) First-use syndrome.

(B) Hypersensitivity.

(C) Pyrogen reaction.

(D) All of the above.

(136) A patient is found in the hemodialysis unit eating food with a non-sterile fork, drinking water, and smoking. What should be strictly prohibited in the dialysis treatment area?

(A) Eating homemade food.

(B) The use of non-sterile silverware.

(C) Drinking water.

(D) Smoking.

(137) A 48-year-old woman is on hemodialysis and her family comes to visit. Her doctor and nurse enter the room to check on the process. Which of these individuals is expected to follow proper hand hygiene protocols?

(A) Healthcare providers.

(B) Patients and their family members.

(C) Only patients.

(D) Options A and B.

(138) In a busy dialysis unit, a 55-year-old patient develops an infection at the catheter site. What step should be taken before the initiation of the disinfection process to prevent further complications?

(A) Administer antibiotics.

(B) Drain the dialysis machine.

(C) Perform mechanical cleaning.

(D) Transfer the patient to another unit.

(139) A staff member is responsible for cleaning the surfaces at the dialysis station. He starts to clean the dialysis chair, countertops, and external surfaces of the dialysis machine. What additional items require mechanical cleaning followed by disinfection?

(A) Medications.

(B) Medical records.

(C) Hemostats and clamps.

(D) Patient's personal belongings.

(140) A technician manages a single-pass dialysis machine for a 70-year-old patient. When should the technician initiate the disinfection process for the machine?

(A) After each use.

(B) At the beginning of each shift.

(C) Whenever visible contamination is present.

(D) Only in the case of a blood leak.

(141) During a dialysis session, the external venous pressure transducer protector becomes wet for a 60-year-old patient. What is the immediate action to ensure safety?

(A) Leave it to dry naturally.

(B) Replace it immediately.

(C) Continue usage with caution.

(D) Disinfect it with alcohol wipes.

(142) A healthcare provider notices bloodline pressure alarms and adjustments of blood drip chamber levels on the dialysis machine during a hemodialysis session for a 45-year-old patient. What could this pattern of alarms and adjustments indicate?

(A) Routine maintenance issue.

(B) A need to replace the pressure protector.

(C) A potential problem with equipment contamination.

(D) An issue with the patient's medical records.

(143) Which of the following dialysis techniques can be performed manually by the patient?

(A) Continuous cycling peritoneal dialysis.

(B) Nightly intermittent peritoneal dialysis.

(C) Continuous ambulatory peritoneal dialysis.

(D) Tidal peritoneal dialysis.

(144) The doctor has recommended that a patient undergoes CAPD. In this technique, the patient or a caregiver instills fluid in the peritoneal cavity. The fluid dwells in the abdominal cavity for a defined period called the dwell period. During the dwell time, what should the patient do?

(A) Remain in bed still.

(B) Move a little as allowed, but with caution.

(C) Stay in the hospital.

(D) Proceed with their regular activities.

(145) How does the permeability of the peritoneal membrane influence the choice of dialysis treatment modality?

(A) It has no effect on the choice of dialysis treatment.

(B) A patient with a more permeable peritoneal membrane should undergo automated peritoneal dialysis.

(C) A patient with a more permeable peritoneal membrane should undergo continuous ambulatory peritoneal dialysis.

(D) A patient with a more permeable peritoneal membrane should not be put on dialysis.

(146) Which of the following contains some of the advantages of APD over CAPD?

(A) Psychosocial benefits include reduced intra-abdominal pressure and lower risk of peritonitis.

(B) It stimulates erythropoietin production from the kidneys, regulates blood pressure, and reduces the risk of glomerulonephritis.

(C) It increases the residual kidney function, reduces abdominal pain, and reduces risk of nephrolithiasis.

(D) It improves the peritoneal membrane structure, improves the residual kidney function, and ameliorates the effects of diabetic nephropathy.

(147) Which dialysis treatment modality is currently the most used in the world?

(A) TPD.

(B) CCPD.

(C) CIPD.

(D) CAPD.

(148) Which of the following is not an issue of CAPD treatment?

(A) Lack of motivation of the patient.

(B) Increased risk of peritonitis.

(C) Failure in technique.

(D) Increased risk of cholelithiasis.

(149) Which of the following is expected to occur after long-term CAPD treatment?

(A) An alteration of glomerulus function.

(B) Alteration in the structure of the peritoneal membrane.

(C) Systemic skin changes.

(D) Reduced cardiovascular compliance.

(150) Which of the following are the most essential factors in deciding a dialysis treatment modality?

(A) Quality of life and patient preference.

(B) Presence of lower back pain and spondylosis.

(C) Education of the patient's family and caretaker.

(D) Presence of comorbidities and treatment for diabetes.

Test 3 Answers and Explanations

(1) (A) Renal fascia.

The microstructure of the kidney includes the nephron and its parts as well as its supporting microstructure. Each healthy human kidney has about 1–1.3 million nephrons. Each nephron consists of the renal corpuscle, the proximal convoluted tubule, the loop of Henle, the distal convoluted tubule, and the collecting ducts.

(2) (B) The renal corpuscle is responsible for the filtration of blood.

The renal corpuscle is formed by the glomerulus and the Bowman capsule. The renal corpuscle is responsible for the filtration of blood through the filtration membrane, which is composed of three layers: the glomerular capillary endothelium, the basement membrane, and the podocyte layer. Blood comes into the glomerulus through the afferent arteriole and leaves through the efferent arteriole.

(3) (D) The primary role of the proximal convoluted tubule is the reabsorption of water and electrolytes.

The proximal convoluted tubule is the coiled initial portion of the nephron that arises from the Bowman capsule and continues as a descending limb of the loop of Henle. It is formed by a layer of cuboidal epithelium that interdigitates and possesses hairlike projections called microvilli. The primary role of the proximal convoluted tubule is for reabsorption of water and electrolytes such as sodium, chloride, calcium, potassium, and bicarbonate from the renal corpuscular filtrate.

(4) (C) Thick distal convoluted tubule.

The Loop of Henle consists of the descending limb, the hairpin bend, and the ascending limb. The descending limb has two segments: the thick descending segment, which is a direct continuation of the proximal convoluted tubule, and the thin descending segments, which are a continuation of the thick descending segment.

(5) (B) It is lined by a layer of cuboidal epithelium called intercalated cells.

The distal convoluted tubule is the continuation of the thick ascending segment of the loop of Henle and continues as the collecting duct. The distal convoluted tubule is about 14–15 mm in length, with a diameter of 22–50 μ. It is lined by a layer of cuboidal epithelium called intercalated cells.

(6) (D) Renin cells.

The juxtaglomerular apparatus is a combination of structures situated near the glomerulus of each nephron. It is formed by the macula densa, the mesangial cells, and the juxtaglomerular cells. The macula densa are cuboidal cells that are aggregated at the terminal portion of thick ascending segment of the loop of Henle, just before opening into the distal convoluted tubule and between the afferent and efferent arterioles.

(7) (D) They are a condensation of cells of the terminal portion of the collecting duct.

Juxtaglomerular cells are smooth muscle cells containing secretory granules within their cytoplasm. It is located within the tunica media and the tunica adventitia of the afferent arteriole shortly before entering the Bowman capsule. The juxtaglomerular apparatus is a combination of structures situated near the glomerulus of each nephron. It is formed by the macula densa, the mesangial cells, and the juxtaglomerular cells.

(8) (A) The juxtaglomerular apparatus secretes hormones, which include renin and prostaglandins.

The juxtaglomerular apparatus secretes hormones such as renin and prostaglandins. It also regulates the glomerular blood flow and the filtration rate. It has no known role in the regulation of vitamin D, erythropoiesis, and thrombopoietin.

(9) (D) Angiotensin is converted to angiotensin I.

The cascade of reactions is stimulated by a fall in arterial blood pressure, reduced extracellular fluid volume, and reduced sodium chloride concentration. Renin catalyzes the conversion of angiotensinogen to angiotensin I, which is physiologically inactive. Angiotensin I is converted to angiotensin II by an angiotensin-converting enzyme produced in the lungs.

(10) (C) It causes constriction of the efferent arteriole, which results in decreased glomerular filtration rate.

Angiotensin II is a potent arteriolar vasoconstrictor that increases blood pressure by vasoconstriction. It also increases the release of noradrenaline from postganglionic sympathetic fibers with resultant increased blood pressure. It acts on the kidneys by causing constriction of the efferent arteriole, which results in the reduction of glomerular filtration rate. It also inhibits the baroreceptor reflex, which is responsible for decreasing the blood.

(11) (B) Membranous nephropathy.

Membranous nephropathy is commonly associated with systemic lupus erythematosus (SLE). It is characterized by immune complex deposition in the glomerular basement membrane, which causes proteinuria and edema.

IgG4-related disease, hemophagocytic conditions, and Henoch Schönlein purpura are not typically associated with SLE-related kidney disease.

(12) (C) Small blood vessels.

Henoch-Schönlein purpura (HSP) is a vasculitis that primarily affects small blood vessels, especially capillaries and postcapillary venules. This condition is characterized by the deposition of immune complexes within these vessels.

(13) (C) Henoch Schönlein purpura.

Henoch Schönlein purpura is a vasculitis mediated by IgA and can cause kidney disease. It is poorly understood but believed to stem from genetic and environmental factors. It is distinct from systemic lupus erythematosus, IgG4-related disease, and hemophagocytic conditions.

(14) (A) PAAN.

A useful mnemonic used to remember the key clinical features of Henoch Schönlein purpura is PAAN – non-blanching purpura, abdominal pain, arthralgia, and nephropathy.

(15) (D) Skin.

The liver, lungs, kidneys, and central nervous system are all impacted by heavy metals. These molecules will deposit in these organs, which precipitates parenchymal damage and organ dysfunction. Although the skin is a common route of exposure to heavy metals, it rarely presents with significant symptoms except for contact eczema.

(16) (A) Protein-bound form.

In chronic exposure to heavy metals, the protein-bound form of heavy metals is generally conjugated by glutathione and metallothionein and gets released into the blood. The ionized form may also contribute to renal damage, but the protein-bound form is significant.

(17) (A) Proximal tubule and loop of Henle.

The proximal tubule and loop of Henle are involved in the reabsorption of ionized metals, which causes acute kidney injury. The distal tubule and collecting duct are not involved in this process.

(18) (A) Shift focus to the patient's lifestyle.

When a patient's kidney disease cannot be attributed to common etiologies, clinicians should consider shifting focus to the patient's lifestyle. This includes assessing for possible exposure to nephrotoxic substances, dietary habits, and other environmental factors.

(19) (B) Podocin gene.

Steroid-resistant nephrotic syndrome due to podocin mutations is an example of a single-gene defect that can cause kidney disease.

Dystrophin is a gene responsible for production of the dystrophin protein, which is indispensable for the function of stria muscles. Mutation of dystrophin causes Duchein's Duchenne muscular dystrophy. CFTR is the gene that causes cystic fibrosis when mutated. The HEXA gene encodes for a subunit of an enzyme called beta-hexosaminidase A. A mutation in the HEXA gene causes Tay-Sachs disease.

(20) (A) Use of targeted drugs.

Future therapy to manage renal disease caused by genetic mutations may involve the development of targeted drugs using gene therapy. This approach holds promise for treating hereditary kidney diseases.

(21) (C) By assessment of albuminuria or other signs of kidney damage.

Patients with stage 1 chronic kidney disease are usually asymptomatic and often have normal or borderline eGFR. The reduction in eGFR may not be overt or sufficient for the diagnosis of CKD at this stage. However, even in the presence of normal eGFR, albuminuria and other signs of kidney damage (such as imaging evidence, histology evidence, and urine sediments) will be present.

(22) (A) To prevent further kidney damage.

The management goal of stage 1 chronic kidney disease is primarily focused on slowing the progression of kidney damage and reduction of risk factors for further kidney impairment.

(23) (C) His ankle edema likely resulted from right-sided heart failure.

His ankle edema is likely due to the kidneys struggling to regulate fluid balance. With an eGFR of 30-59 mL/min/1.73m^2, this man is in stage 3 CKD. Hyperphosphatemia is a common complication of CKD. Management and treatment of stage 3 CKD is essential and should aim to slow disease progression, manage symptoms, and address complications.

(24) (B) Stage 2.

ACR is based on the severity of proteinuria in the form of urinary albumin levels. ACR and urinary albumin excretion over 24 hours can classify CKD as follows:

- A1: ACR less than 3 mg/mmol or albumin excretion less than 30 mg/24hr.
- A2: ACR 3-30 mg/mmol or albumin excretion 30-300 mg/24hr.
- A3: ACR greater than 30 mg/mmol or albumin excretion greater than 300 mg/24hr.

(25) (C) 1 and 2.

CKD can be classified according to the eGFR category, albumin-creatinine ratio, and albumin excretion. Another way of classifying CKD is according to the cause of etiology.

(26) (C) Three months.

The guideline for defining chronic kidney disease is kidney damage or a decreased glomerular filtration rate of less than 60 mL/min/1.73m2 for at least three months. Evidence of kidney damage may include microalbuminuria, urine sediments, and histological and imaging abnormalities.

(27) (A) Increase the Epoetin alfa dosage.

The severity of anemia in CKD is directly related to the extent of kidney function loss because the kidneys play a crucial role in erythropoiesis. Patients with chronic kidney disease have a primary deficiency in erythropoietin production by interstitial cells of the kidneys. Thus, erythropoietin dosage must be adjusted until a satisfactory hemoglobin level is obtained. This patient is anemic and the erythropoietin dosage has to be increased.

(28) (C) Urinary loss of complement proteins.

Patients with CKD are more likely to have infections due to the loss of complement proteins in the urine.

(29) (C) 15-29 mL/min/1.73m^2.

In stage 4 CKD, there is a severe reduction in eGFR with values as low as 15-29 mL/min/1.73m^2.

(30) (B) Stage 1.

In stage 1 chronic kidney disease, the eGFR is usually greater than or equal to 90 mL/min/1.73m^2 (normal or elevated eGFR value). This stage indicates that kidney function is still relatively normal. However, there may be signs of renal damage, such as proteinuria.

(31) (B) Metabolic alkalosis.

Metabolic alkalosis is not usually associated with CKD, but it is seen in conditions associated with excessive vomiting or excessive use of bicarbonate. Hyperkalemia, osteoporosis, and anemia are common complications seen in patients with CKD.

(32) (C) Benign prostatic hyperplasia.

Benign prostatic hyperplasia is a benign disorder in which the enlarged prostate gland causes postrenal AKI as it narrows and obstructs the flow of urine out of the urinary bladder. This results in increased intraluminal pressure, which thereby impairs urine flow. Acute tubular necrosis, acute interstitial nephritis, and glomerulonephritis are common causes of intrarenal AKI.

(33) (C) Ibuprofen.

Ibuprofen is an NSAID that should be avoided in patients with AKI because it can potentially worsen kidney function. NSAIDs can cause renal vasoconstriction and thus reduce GFR. Amoxicillin, acetaminophen, and diphenhydramine are generally considered safe for patients with AKI, although their dosages may need to be adjusted.

(34) (C) Kidney transplantation.

The GFR range seen in ESKD (5–10 mL/min/1.73m^2) indicates an extremely limited kidney function. At this stage, the kidneys cannot effectively filter waste products or regulate fluid and electrolyte balance. This results in the buildup of toxins in the body. In this scenario, renal replacement therapy becomes necessary to take over the role of the kidneys. The three modalities for renal replacement therapy are kidney transplantation, hemodialysis, and peritoneal dialysis. Kidney transplantation is considered the most effective option of renal replacement therapy because it improves the quality of life, provides a chance for long-term survival, eliminates dialysis dependence, improves cardiovascular health and nutritional status, and reduces uremic symptoms.

(35) (A) The stage of CKD.

Understanding the stages of CKD is necessary to assess prognosis and determine appropriate management strategies. In the early stages (one through three), the kidney function is mildly to moderately impaired, and lifestyle adjustments and proper management play an important role in slowing down or halting the disease's progression. In advanced stages (four and five), kidney function is severely impaired, and the prognosis is worrisome. Even with aggressive management, the progression to ESKD is likely for these patients.

(36) (C) To improve the quality of life and long-term survival in patients with CKD.

Renal replacement therapy is a critical intervention for individuals with ESKD. It is not only a life-sustaining intervention but a comprehensive attempt to improve the patient's quality of life, alleviate distressing symptoms, reduce the risk of complications, and create the possibility of an extended and fulfilling life.

(37) (D) To prevent further deterioration and restore function.

The primary objective is based on the understanding that AKI is usually reversible, especially when diagnosed and treated promptly and appropriately. Healthcare providers can give patients the best chance at recovery and long-term health through targeted, individualized care.

(38) (B) Significant decline in the glomerular filtration rate.

The main indication for kidney transplants in patients with End-Stage Kidney Disease is a significant decline in the glomerular filtration rate, which indicates a severe loss of kidney function. GFR is a critical measure of kidney function, and a substantial reduction in GFR signifies that the kidneys are no longer able to effectively filter waste products from the blood. This decline in kidney function is a key criterion for considering kidney transplants as a treatment option, as it typically indicates that the patient has reached a stage where dialysis or transplant is necessary to sustain life.

(39) (B) Renal artery thrombosis.

Prerenal AKI is a type of kidney injury that occurs due to external factors that cause a reduction in blood flow to the kidneys, which impairs their ability to filter and excrete waste products. Renal artery thrombosis is an example of a condition that can cause prerenal AKI. The thrombus occludes the flow of oxygenated blood in the renal artery to the kidney, and the affected kidney receives less blood supply, which, in severe cases, can result in prerenal AKI.

(40) (B) Control protein intake.

Dietary management is an important component in the overall care of individuals with CKD as it helps slow the disease's progression and manage complications associated with impaired kidney function. Control of protein intake is a form of dietary management required for patients with CKD. Proteins are essential nutrients needed for tissue repair, enzyme production, and regulation of immune function. When CKD compromises the kidneys, their ability to effectively process and excrete the byproducts of protein metabolism is reduced. Dietary management requires high-quality protein sources that are easily processed by the kidneys, e.g., lean meats, poultry, fish, and dairy products. Patients may be advised to limit their intake of high-protein foods such as red meats and certain beans.

(41) (B) Hypermagnesemia

Hypermagnesemia is seen with impaired capability of the kidney to maintain a state of electrolyte balance with progression of the disease.

(42) (B) Rapid breathing.

Rapid breathing is a respiratory compensation mechanism to correct acid-base imbalances. This can be a sign of compensation in kidney disease patients with acidosis.

(43) (A) Potassium restriction.

Potassium restriction is the appropriate measure to be taken as the other available measures would lead to other imbalances.

(44) (C) Decreased absorption of calcium due to impaired vitamin D activation.

The kidneys activate vitamin D. When they are not functioning properly, vitamin D is not activated and calcium absorption is decreased.

(45) (D) Consumption of bananas and oranges.

Consumption of bananas and oranges will further raise the potassium levels. Max has to avoid them to help keep the levels moderate.

(46) (B) Hypertension causes a progressive fall in kidney function in chronic kidney disease patients.

Hypertension is believed to contribute to the acceleration of progressive decline in kidney function as seen in patients with CKD. This includes the risk for CVD and associated mortality.

(47) (B) Swelling in the feet and legs.

Hypernatremia is characterized by excess sodium in the body and can cause fluid retention, which is a common issue in patients with CKD. This fluid retention often manifests as swelling or edema in the feet and legs.

(48) (A) Anemia is found in 50% of patients with advanced chronic kidney disease.

In CKD patients, anemia begins early in the course of the disease and becomes more severe as viable kidney mass decreases and glomerular filtration rate gradually declines. Information from the National Health and Nutrition Examination Survey show that anemia is twice as common in people with chronic kidney disease than in the general population and more than half of patients with advanced chronic kidney disease have anemia.

(49) (D) Mineral and bone disorders may present risk of premature death in chronic kidney disease patients as well as increased risk for cardiovascular disease and its associated complications.

Chronic renal failure is often complicated by abnormal bone and mineral ion homeostasis. This may contribute to the accelerated development of cardiovascular disease. Therefore, mineral and bone diseases are identified as risk factors for premature death and cardiovascular diseases in CKD patients. Skeletal and extra-skeletal complications, which may include abnormalities in bone remodeling, mineralization, or linear growth, as well as vascular or soft tissue calcification, are commonly observed in patients with chronic kidney disease. Because of the increased incidence of osteoporosis and osteoporotic fractures in patients with chronic kidney disease, vitamin D is recommended in the early stages of the disease.

(50) (B) Every 6 months.

Cardiovascular risk should be assessed regularly in CKD patients, ideally every 6 months, due to their increased risk of cardiovascular disease and the non-specific nature of related signs and symptoms. Regular assessment helps in early identification and management of cardiovascular issues.

(51) (D) Hypocalcemia.

Hypocalcemia can cause symptoms like confusion, muscle cramps, and cardiac arrhythmias. Since the potassium levels are near normal, hypocalcemia is a likely cause of these symptoms in a chronic kidney disease patient.

(52) (B) Congestive heart failure.

The patient has chronic kidney disease-related hypertension (fluid overload) which has led to the development of heart failure. This can also result from electrolyte abnormalities. Congestive heart failure is a prevalent cardiovascular consequence in people with chronic kidney disease, especially when it is severe.

(53) (D) Atrial fibrillation.

Patients with CKD frequently experience atrial fibrillation and especially those who have a history of hypertension. Chronic kidney disease can cause structural cardiac abnormalities and electrolyte imbalances, which increase the risk of atrial fibrillation.

(54) (C) Altered bone metabolism and remodeling.

Renal osteodystrophy is a mineral and bone disorder commonly associated with CKD. It is characterized by altered bone metabolism and remodeling. Due to the kidneys' impaired function in CKD, they are less efficient in maintaining the balance of minerals such as calcium and phosphorus, and in producing active vitamin D. These disturbances lead to various bone problems, including changes in bone structure, density, and strength.

(55) (D) Hypertension.

The left ventricle becomes hypertrophied in the process of pumping out blood at high pressure into the systemic circulation. It thickens with time.

(56) (B) Uremic pericarditis

Uremic pericarditis is mostly prevalent in patients with advanced kidney disease. Symptoms include chest pain that intensifies during inhalation, a distinctive pericardial friction sound when listening to the heart, and specific changes that are observed on an ECG.

(57) (C) There is no clear underlying risk factor for the anuria.

Acute anuria, or the complete absence of urine output, can be a symptom of various underlying conditions. In the absence of a clear underlying risk factor, it is not an immediate indication for a renal biopsy in a young patient. A renal biopsy is an invasive procedure generally reserved for when there is a suspicion of specific kidney diseases that can be diagnosed or ruled out by examining kidney tissue. In cases where there are no evident risk factors or causes of acute anuria, other diagnostic methods and assessments are usually considered before proceeding to a renal biopsy.

(58) (C) Anti-GBM disease.

Anti-GBM disease is characterized by crescentic glomerulonephritis in the light microscope and linear deposition of IgG on glomerular capillaries in the electron microscope.

(59) (B) Lupus nephritis.

Lupus nephritis is characterized by thickening of the GBM mesangial expansion, endothelial cell swelling, podocyte foot process effacement, and full house immunofluorescence.

(60) (A) Increased creatinine of >10.

Indications for initiating patients on dialysis include uremic symptoms, refractory hyperkalemia, refractory academia, refractory fluid overload, bleeding diathesis, and GFR less than 10. Creatinine by itself is not enough to assess whether a patient requires dialysis.

(61) (D) Peritonitis.

Hypotension, nonfunctional hemodialysis access, and anaphylactic reactions to the dialysate are all possible complications of hemodialysis. Peritonitis is a common complication of peritoneal dialysis.

(62) (D) Induction immunosuppressive therapy is given long-term to prevent rejection.

Induction therapy is given immediately after rejection and maintenance immunotherapy is given long-term.

(63) (C) Stop all nephrotoxic medications.

In this case of contrast-induced nephrotoxicity, the creatinine increased but is still less than 2.5 times the baseline. The next step would be to stop any further nephrotoxic insults and monitor creatinine. Kidney biopsy and dialysis are not indicated.

(64) (B) Angiotensinogen.

Erythropoietin, prostaglandins, and renin are produced by the kidney as a secretory function. Angiotensinogen is produced by the liver.

(65) (A) Renal ultrasound.

In chronic kidney disease, ultrasound can show an increased signal in the renal cortex and a loss of distinction between the cortex and medulla. It can also show a decrease in renal size.

(66) (B) Blood pressure.

Blood pressure is monitored very closely after kidney biopsy to detect bleeding early. Hypotension can indicate hemorrhage.

(67) (A) Conventional hemodialysis.

Conventional hemodialysis is associated with interdialytic fluid accumulation due to the longer interval of dialysis sessions. The fluid has enough time to build up before the next dialysis session.

(68) (C) Short daily home dialysis.

This modality best describes Mr. Y's dialysis schedule, which he does at home.

(69) (D) Conventional hemodialysis.

There is an increased need for antihypertensive medications in conventional dialysis. The abnormal blood pressure could cause cardiac complications if care is not taken.

(70) (B) Conventional hemodialysis.

Conventional hemodialysis uses low-flux dialyzers. These have a low permeability for water and filter at a slower rate.

(71) (C) Each session is shorter, but they occur more frequently.

In short daily dialysis, the aim is to filter toxins as close to the natural kidney function as possible. Thus, the procedure is done many days within the week.

(72) (B) From a region of high concentration to a region of low concentration.

Diffusion is the process whereby molecules move from an area of higher concentration to an area of lower concentration, which is a fundamental principle in dialysis for removing waste products from the blood.

(73) (C) At the center by the patient.

In this type of hemodialysis, the patient goes to the dialysis center. However, they are responsible for administering treatment themselves.

(74) (C) Heightened risk of vascular access complications.

This is not an advantage but rather a disadvantage of short daily dialysis.

(75) (A) Convection only.

Only convection is used in hemofiltration. Convection refers to the transport of both the solute and solvent across a semipermeable membrane.

(76) (A) The inflexible schedule.

This is unlike home dialysis, which is flexible and based on the patient's preference.

(77) (D) Steal syndrome.

Steal syndrome happens when arterial inflow becomes restricted and flow through the fistula or graft is less resistant than other distal vascular beds. In extreme circumstances, it could result in digital gangrene.

(78) (C) Central venous catheter.

Central venous catheter is a type of temporary percutaneous access and should be used when access is required for less than three weeks. It is primarily used in cases where emergency or urgent hemodialysis is warranted. This immediate measure is often employed at the onset of renal replacement therapy, in scenarios where the long-term access is rendered dysfunctional, or in instances where a brief period of hemodialysis treatment is necessitated.

(79) (A) Ultrasound and x-ray.

An ultrasound is used to guide the insertion of a central venous catheter. An x-ray is used to confirm the placement.

(80) (C) Central venous catheter.

A central venous catheter carries the highest risk of infection and needs continuous checking. It should not stay in place for more than three weeks.

(81) (B) Bruit.

A stethoscope placed in AVF is to auscultate for bruit, a turbulent blood flow in AVF. A healthy AV fistula has a bruit.

(82) (B) Regularly wash catheter exits with clean water and soap.

Catheter sites should be dry at all times. Patients should avoid exposing the site to water during activities and use a waterproof dressing before bathing.

(83) (C) Central venous catheter.

In every patient with a central venous catheter in situ, it is important to rule out catheter-associated infections as they are more serious and likely.

(84) (C) Thrill or bruit.

Patient education is vital for maintaining the functionality and health of the AVF/AVG. Patients should regularly check for thrill or bruit, avoid constrictive clothing, heavy loads on the affected arm, and extreme temperatures.

(85) (C) Adequate flushing and heparin lock.

Blockage is a common problem with catheters, which can cause reduced flow rates and ineffective dialysis. Adequate flushing of the catheter and using a heparin lock can often prevent this issue.

(86) (C) Radiocephalic.

In that order, the preferred locations for AVF are radiocephalic, radiobasilic, brachiocephalic, and brachiobasilic transposition.

(87) (B) Polysulfone.

Polysulfone is the primary material used in modern dialyzer membranes in the United States. It is a biocompatible synthetic membrane material used to make dialyzer membranes.

(88) (B) 136–140 mmol/L.

The standard range for dialysate sodium concentration during hemodialysis is 136–140 mmol/L. This range helps maintain electrolyte balance.

(89) (B) To counterbalance urea-related osmolar gradients.

Sodium modeling may counterbalance urea-related osmolar gradients, especially in patients who frequently experience hypotension during dialysis. It gradually reduces dialysate sodium concentration to mitigate these gradients.

(90) (B) To maintain a balanced electrolyte profile.

The primary purpose of adjustment of the composition of the dialysate solution is to maintain a balanced electrolyte profile during dialysis and maintain electrolyte levels within a safe range.

(91) (D) Reverse osmosis.

Water used for dialysate undergoes treatment, which includes reverse osmosis, to eliminate microbiological contaminants and dissolved ions, which ensures its purity for use in hemodialysis.

(92) (C) Blood Pressure.

Blood pressure monitoring is the most important vital sign during dialysis. Blood pressure fluctuations can have a significant impact on the patient during dialysis. Hypotension or hypertension are severe complications that can arise from hemodialysis. These complications are due to rapid changes in fluid levels during dialysis. Hence, maintenance of optimal blood pressure is an essential step in hemodialysis. In addition, the long-term benefits of hemodialysis are linked with an optimal blood pressure reading.

(93) (C) Dehydration.

Dehydration occurs when fluid removal exceeds normal during dialysis. It is also another complication of hemodialysis. When excess fluid is filtered out during dialysis, dehydration occurs. Dehydration during dialysis can present in many ways, such as low blood pressure, dizziness, and muscle cramps. It can also cause cardiovascular problems during dialysis. Close monitoring during dialysis will ensure proper hydration for the patient.

(94) (A) Vital Signs.

Patient monitoring is achieved through the assessment of vital signs. The patient's vital signs are a significant indicator of complications. They also indicate the patient's tolerance of the procedure. These vital signs include blood pressure, respiratory rate, heart rate, temperature, and oxygen saturation. Any possible complication would reflect on the patient's vital signs. Hence, it is essential to monitor vital signs during dialysis.

(95) (A) To prevent excessive bleeding.

Anticoagulation monitoring is essential during hemodialysis to prevent excessive bleeding within the dialysis circuit and maintain uninterrupted blood flow and treatment efficacy.

(96) (C) Cleaning and disinfection protocols.

In facilities where dialyzers are reused, stringent cleaning and disinfection protocols help to prevent contamination-related complications.

(97) (D) Fistula and Graft.

Hemodialysis access is also called vascular access. Vascular access allows blood flow to the dialysis machine. The dialyzer filters the blood through ultrafiltration. Vascular access occurs through a minor surgical procedure. The methods of vascular access include a fistula, a graft, or a catheter. A fistula is usually the first choice. However, a graft or catheter method is primary if blood vessels are not strong enough.

(98) (A) Dialysate.

The dialysate is responsible for filtration of waste from the blood. It works through diffusion. The dialysate solution is individualized for each patient in accordance with their needs. It creates a concentration gradient through which waste products flow into it from the blood. Hence, it performs the function of the kidneys while inside the dialyzer. It maintains the body's electrolyte balance while filtering waste.

(99) (B) Higher blood flow increases efficacy.

A higher blood flow rate increases the efficiency of the dialyzer during dialysis. A high blood flow rate would allow more waste to filter into the dialysate. The removal of adequate waste is the aim of dialysis. Therefore, increasing the flow rate of blood increases efficiency. However, one must be careful to prevent complications. The patient's requirements must be considered during dialysis.

(100) (C) Pre-dialysis evaluation.

The first step in monitoring the hemodialysis process is the pre-dialysis evaluation, which includes assessment of the patient's medical history, physical condition, and laboratory tests to tailor the treatment plan.

(101) (A) High-flux dialyzer.

High-flux dialyzers are designed to clear large molecules efficiently. Their membranes have large pores, which makes them suitable for patients with high molecular weight toxins like beta 2-microglobulin.

(102) (B) To minimize biocompatibility-related reactions.

Highly permeable dialyzers are usually made with synthetic membranes, and are designed to minimize biocompatibility-related reactions. These reactions occur when the body's immune system reacts to the dialyzer membrane, which can cause complications such as inflammation and reduced dialysis efficiency. Synthetic membranes are engineered to be more biocompatible, which reduces the likelihood of these immune responses.

(103) (D) Parallel plate dialyzer.

Parallel plate dialyzers have a compact design, which makes them space-efficient without sacrificing filtering capacity or biocompatibility.

(104) (D) Hollow fiber dialyzer.

Hollow fiber dialyzers have a membrane barrier between the blood and the dialysate. This minimizes the likelihood of blood contamination or leakage into the dialysate.

(105) (C) They effectively remove both small and midsized solutes.

High-flux dialyzers are preferred in certain hemodialysis treatments because they effectively remove both small solutes and midsized solutes. This efficacy is due to their larger pore size and increased permeability. The larger pores allow for more efficient clearance of midsized molecules, such as beta-2 microglobulin, which are not as effectively removed by low-flux dialyzers with smaller pores.

(106) (D) An anticoagulant such as heparin.

Heparin is the substance used during dialysis to prevent blood from clotting as it moves through the dialysis machine. While heparin is not a physical component of the machine itself, it's integral to the dialysis process, often added to the blood circuit or delivery system to maintain a clot-free environment. The blood pump, dialyzer, and control panel are parts of the machine that manage the flow and filtration of blood, but they do not have intrinsic anticoagulant properties.

(107) (B) Three times per week.

This patient should receive dialysis thrice weekly, for three to six hours per session.

(108) (A) Potassium.

During dialysis, potassium levels can rise and cause hyperkalemia. Patients should consume potassium in strict moderation to prevent this.

(109) (C) To manage the patient's electrolyte balance.

Potassium is an essential electrolyte that must be carefully managed in patients undergoing hemodialysis. In the dialysis process, the concentration of potassium in the dialysate is meticulously controlled and adjusted to manage the patient's electrolyte balance.

(110) (B) The urea concentration.

Urea concentration is a waste product that must be filtered completely out of blood and, therefore, cannot be part of the dialysate.

(111) (D) Calcium chloride ($CaCl_2$).

Calcium, in the form of calcium chloride, is included in the dialysate solution used in hemodialysis to prevent the loss of calcium from patients who undergo the treatment.

(112) (A) Bicarbonate (HCO_3^-).

Bicarbonate buffers acidosis in the blood during hemodialysis. End products from the reaction of bicarbonate and excess hydrogen ions are easy to clear. Therefore, the blood's acidity is reduced.

(113) (B) To provide a source of energy for the patient.

Glucose is added to dialysate to prevent hypoglycemia and serve as an energy source (because it can be utilized by the cells during the hemodialysis process)

(114) (A) To reduce costs.

Reusing dialyzers reduces costs in budget-limited facilities. Highly sterile measures should be taken to prevent infections

(115) (B) They are subjected to a thorough cleaning and disinfection process.

Dialyzers are thoroughly cleaned, disinfected, and sterilized before reuse.

(116) (B) Muscle cramps.

Chest pain is a prominent complaint in angina, myocardial infarction, and air embolism.

(117) (D) It is the presence of air in the lungs and systemic circulation.

Air embolism is the presence of air into an extracorporeal system that spreads into systemic circulation.

(118) (D) All of the above.

Clinical features of air embolism include a pink foamy air pocket in the extracorporeal system venous line, cough, shortness of breath, chest pain or pressure, tachycardia, distended neck veins, cyanosis, confusion, convulsions, coma, and possible cardio-respiratory arrest.

(119) (C) Loosen connections when priming.

Prevention of air embolism includes keeping the level of drip chambers up, replacing empty saline bags immediately, and tightening connections when priming.

(120) (A) Muscle cramps and twitching.

Features of hypocalcemia include muscle cramps, spasms, numbness, tingling sensations, and tetany or seizures.

(121) (A) Excess removal of fluid.

Hypotension often results from the rapid removal of excess fluids during hemodialysis, and it is the primary mechanism behind intradialysis hypotension.

(122) (B) Clotting.

Anticoagulation is a treatment modality that is used for conditions related to clotting. Medications are used to help prevent blood clots from forming or growing larger.

Anticoagulation therapy is used in conditions like deep vein thrombosis, pulmonary embolism, and in some cases of atrial fibrillation.

(123) (C) Release of intracellular potassium.

The breakdown or destruction of red blood cells releases potassium from the damaged cells into the bloodstream, which causes hyperkalemia.

(124) (D) All of the above.

The etiology of hemolysis in hemodialysis patients is usually related to multiple causes. This includes poorly functioning or incorrectly calibrated blood pump, excessive negative pressure in the extracorporeal circuit, deformity in lines, and overocclusion of the blood pump.

(125) (C) Chest pain.

Dialysis disequilibrium syndrome is characterized by neurological symptoms rather than cardiac symptoms. It is a rare but serious complication of hemodialysis, particularly in patients who are new to dialysis or those with severe uremia. Common symptoms include headache, nausea, restlessness, and in more severe cases, altered mental status and seizures. These symptoms result from cerebral edema and the rapid changes in the brain's osmotic gradient during dialysis. Chest pain is not typically a symptom of dialysis disequilibrium syndrome.

(126) (B) Elevated levels of parathyroid hormone due to primary hyperparathyroidism.

Itching (pruritus) in dialyzed patients can often be attributed to primary hyperparathyroidism, which is a condition that leads to elevated levels of parathyroid hormone. High PTH levels can result from the impaired renal function associated with kidney disease, as the kidneys play a vital role in regulating PTH levels. Elevated PTH can affect the skin and cause itching.

(127) (B) Use of short-acting antihypertensives within 4 hours of dialysis.

The use of short-acting antihypertensives within 4 hours of hemodialysis, especially vasodilators, results in the development of hypotension during hemodialysis.

(128) (D) All of the above.

Extreme blood loss in hemodialysis is caused by blood line separation, needles dislodging from access, rupture of anastomosis or aneurysm, crack in dialyzer casing/rupture of dialyzer, and loose dialyzer caps/connections.

(129) (D) Both A and B.

First-use syndrome and hypersensitivity to membrane are forms of dialyzer reactions. Urticaria and pruritis are clinical features of dialyzer reactions.

(130) (B) It usually occurs during the first use of a dialyzer.

First-use syndrome typically occurs during the first use of a new dialyzer or blood tubing set. It is characterized by an allergic reaction, not necessarily reproducible in subsequent sessions and doesn't have to be severe IgE anaphylactoid in nature.

(131) (C) Dialyzer reactions.

The clinical features of hives, angioedema, urticaria, and pruritus are indicative of dialyzer reactions. These reactions can occur in patients who undergo hemodialysis and are allergic to the dialyzer membrane or other components that are used in the dialysis process.

(132) (C) Both A and B.

Causes of hypertension during hemodialysis may include fluid overload, noncompliance with blood pressure medications, anxiety, and renin overproduction.

(133) (C) Treatment with epinephrine and steroids.

To manage a dialyzer reaction, you need to stop the dialysis and then give epinephrine and steroids for anaphylactic reactions and symptomatic management.

(134) (D) All of the above.

Management involves adequate dialysis to regulate electrolyte levels, lotions or medications for dry skin/allergies, and control of uremia and secondary hyperparathyroidism.

(135) (C) Pyrogen reaction.

A pyrogenic reaction is a febrile reaction due to presence of dead bacteria and/or endotoxins within the systemic circulation.

(136) (D) Smoking.

To maintain a sterile environment in the dialysis treatment area, smoking should be strictly prohibited. Smoking introduces contaminants and compromises the safety of both patients and staff. Eating with non-sterile silverware and drinking water can be allowed.

(137) (D) Options A and B.

In the context of infection control in hemodialysis, healthcare providers, patients, and their family members are all supposed to follow proper hand hygiene protocols before entering the dialysis room. This comprehensive approach to hand hygiene is essential for infection control. Unfortunately, family members may not follow these guidelines appropriately, which compromises the sterility of the patient's station.

(138) (C) Perform mechanical cleaning.

Before initiating the disinfection process, it's vital to perform mechanical cleaning. This ensures that surfaces and equipment are free from debris and contaminants. The first option is incorrect because though antibiotics are indeed necessary to treat patients, they are not beneficial in the cleaning process. The second option suggests the draining of the dialysis machine. This is not recommended in most cleansing protocols. The fourth option is clearly a distractor since the transfer of the patient is the opposite of what should be done.

(139) (C) Hemostats and clamps.

Even though cleaning the dialysis chair, countertops, and external surfaces of the dialysis machine is indispensable, certain medical equipment, such as the hemostats and clamps, should also undergo mechanical cleaning since they come into contact with patients. These items can potentially host microbes. Therefore, thorough cleaning and disinfection are necessary. The first, second, and fourth options are incorrect.

(140) (A) After each use.

The disinfection process for a single-pass dialysis machine should be initiated after each use. This practice ensures that the machine is clean and free from potential contaminants for each patient, thereby reducing the risk of infection.

(141) (B) Replace it immediately.

If the external venous pressure transducer protector becomes wet during dialysis, the immediate action is to replace it. Wet protectors can introduce potential contamination and replacement is necessary to maintain aseptic conditions. Leaving the transducer protector to dry will still harbor all sorts of microbes, whereas cautious use is contraindicated. The use of alcohol wipes may not effectively address the contamination.

(142) (C) A potential problem with equipment contamination.

Frequent bloodline pressure alarms and adjustments of blood drip chamber levels may indicate a potential problem with equipment contamination. This pattern suggests that there may be issues with the sterility of the equipment. The first option is incorrect because the alarms and adjustments are not related to routine maintenance.

(143) (C) Continuous ambulatory peritoneal dialysis.

CAPD is a home-based dialysis treatment modality that can be performed by the patient manually. The patient performs the exchange procedure by filling the abdominal cavity with a dialysate that remains there for a dwell period, and then drained out into a bag. The exchange procedure takes around 30 minutes, and the patient performs 3–5 exchanges per day and one during the night.

(144) (D) Proceed with their regular activities.

A patient who is undergoing CAPD can proceed with their regular activities. One of the big advantages of CAPD is that it can be done at any clean and dry place, which allows patient mobility.

(145) (B) A patient with a more permeable peritoneal membrane should undergo automated peritoneal dialysis.

Patients with a more permeable peritoneal membrane have a higher speed of solute and fluid transport from the peritoneum. They are called high transporters. Automated peritoneal dialysis is the preferred choice for high transporters due to its shorter dwell times.

(146) (A) Psychosocial benefits include reduced intra-abdominal pressure and lower risk of peritonitis.

APD allows the patient to have freedom from intra-abdominal fluids during the day, which makes it preferable for patients who are active or working. Because it is done in the supine position during the night, it reduces the intra-abdominal pressure compared to CAPD, which is done in the upright position. It is also associated with a reduced risk of peritonitis because the patient does not have that much contact with the bag.

(147) (D) CAPD.

Continuous Ambulatory Peritoneal Dialysis is currently the most used dialysis treatment modality worldwide due to its flexibility and feasibility for patients to manage at home.

(148) (D) Increased risk of cholelithiasis.

Increased risk of cholelithiasis is not an issue of CAPD treatment because CAPD does not affect the biliary system.

(149) (B) Alteration in the structure of the peritoneal membrane.

CAPD treatment has been shown to alter the peritoneal membrane's structure and function. This may occur due to the recurrence of peritonitis and exposure to high concentrations of glucose, which is contained in the solute. Some structural changes may include submesothelial fibrosis, an increase in fibroblasts, and loss of mesothelial cells.

(150) (A) Quality of life and patient preference.

Patients with active lifestyles, children, workers, and elderly patients prefer APD over CAPD because they are free from intraabdominal fluid during the day. Patient preference increases compliance.

References

1. Barello, S., Anderson, G., Acampora, M., Bosio, C., Guida, E., Irace, V., Guastoni, C. M., Bertani, B., & Graffigna, G. (2023). The effect of psychosocial interventions on depression, anxiety, and quality of life in hemodialysis patients: a systematic review and a meta-analysis. International urology and nephrology, 55(4), 897–912.
2. Borg, R., Carlson, N., Søndergaard, J., & Persson, F. (2023). The Growing Challenge of Chronic Kidney Disease: An Overview of Current Knowledge. International Journal of Nephrology, 2023.
3. By Heidi Noels, Joachim Jankowski Year: 2023 Container: Circulation Research Volume: 132 Issue: 8 Page: 899-901.
4. Dialyzers, dialysate, and delivery systems - Review of Hemodialysis for Nurses and Dialysis Personnel, 8th Edition. (n.d.).
5. Fadem, S. et al (2023). Complications in Dialysis: A Clinical Guide. Springer.
6. Finnigan, N. A., & Leslie, S. W. (2023). Polycystic kidney disease in adults. In StatPearls [Internet]. StatPearls Publishing.
7. Hashmi, Muhammad F., Onecia Benjamin, and Sarah L. Lappin. 2023. "End-Stage Renal Disease." StatPearls, February.
8. Kazi, A. M., & Hashmi, M. F. (2023). Glomerulonephritis. In StatPearls. StatPearls Publishing.
9. Kim, I. S., Kim, S., Yoo, T., & Kim, J. (2023). Diagnosis and management of hypertensive disease in dialysis patients: a systematic review. Clinical Hypertension, 29(1).
10. Nesheiwat, Z., & Lee, J. J. (2023, July 17). Uremic Pericarditis. In: StatPearls [Internet]. Treasure Island (FL): StatPearls Publishing.
11. Sam, R. (n.d.). Hemodialysis: Diffusion and Ultrafiltration.
12. Turgut, F., Awad, A. S., & Abdel-Rahman, E. M. (2023). Acute kidney injury: Medical causes and pathogenesis. Journal of Clinical Medicine, 12(1), 375.

13. Vaglio, A., Gattorno, M., McAdoo, S., Obici, L. P., & Ghiggeri, G. M. (2023). Editorial: The kidney in auto-immune and auto-inflammatory processes: Definitions, mechanisms, and biomarkers. Frontiers in medicine, 9, 1129021.
14. Yeung, A., Aziz, A., Taji, L., Cooper, R., Oliver, M. J., Blake, P. G., & McFarlane, P. (2023). Infection Control Practices in In-Center Hemodialysis Units During Wave 1 of the COVID-19 Pandemic in Ontario, Canada: Research Letter. Canadian journal of kidney health and disease, 10, 20543581221146033.

Made in United States
North Haven, CT
10 November 2026

22097458R00222